Last
VOYAGES

Making Waves

The real lives of sporting heroes on, in & under the water

Also in this series...

Golden Lily
by Lijia Xu
The fascinating autobiography from
Asia's first dinghy sailing gold medallist

The First Indian
by Dilip Donde
The story of the first Indian solo
circumnavigation under sail

more to follow

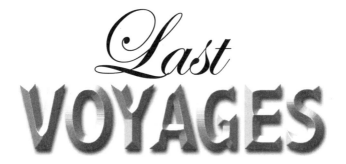

Last VOYAGES

Nicholas Gray

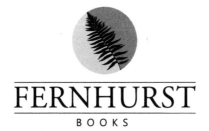

FERNHURST
BOOKS

First published in 2017 by Fernhurst Books Limited
62 Brandon Parade, Holly Walk, Leamington Spa, Warwickshire, CV32 4JE, UK
Tel: +44 (0) 1926 337488 | www.fernhurstbooks.com

A catalogue record for this book is available from the British Library
ISBN 978-1-909911-55-0

Front cover photograph: Philip Walwyn's *Kate* between the English Harbour Heads:
From the Walwyn family archive. By kind permission of Kate Walwyn, Susie Walwyn
and John Halsey.
Back cover photograph: Nicholas Gray: By kind permission of Lester Barnes.

Designed & typeset by Rachel Atkins
Printed in the UK by Clays Ltd, St Ives plc

To Josephine

"Qui vit sans follie
n'est pas aussi sage
qu'il croit"

(author unknown)

Inscription seen by Peter Tangvald
on an ashtray in his parent's house

*"Whoever lives without folly
is not as wise as he thinks"*

Contents

Foreword

by Sir Chay Blyth

No sailor ever embarks on a last voyage. They set out with hopes and aspirations; excitement and perhaps a little apprehension; the horizon offering many possibilities. None of the voyages described in this book were undertaken with the intention of it being the last. But these remarkable sailors all lost their lives at sea, many alone, and many of whose bodies were never returned to land.

In few cases does tragedy occur right away. Often it is significantly into the voyage, in many cases near its completion, when something goes wrong and disaster strikes. Whether through a medical emergency… bad weather… a fault with the vessel… or merely slipping overboard… all of these voyages were their last; although we cannot always be certain exactly what happened.

Nicholas Gray describes, with an elegance and sympathy rightfully deserved by such characters, the lives, sailing careers and final voyages of a number of well-known yachtsmen, all friends of or known to him. He gives a wonderful insight into the people behind the headlines and their lives before the tragedies. This is an excellent tribute to truly great sailors.

Many of those described in this book I have had the pleasure to sail with or compete against. Reading their stories brings them to life again, allowing one to look back and remember their achievements, and enabling their legacy to live on beyond their momentous final voyage.

Last Voyages is a superb read. I thoroughly recommend it for anyone, like me, with a love of the sea or an admiration of those who have the courage to contend with this mighty force of nature.

Introduction

Some years ago whilst on a climbing trip in North Wales, one member of our party said that he was giving up climbing as he knew too many people who had died on the mountains.

I mulled this over during the rest of that weekend. Whilst I had never climbed outside the United Kingdom, I had met or come across several famous climbers in the hills of Scotland and North Wales and I knew that some of them were no longer with us. This was perhaps inevitable as, with every passing year, climbers were taking more and more risks on more and more extreme climbs in more and more severe weather.

Later, lying comfortably in my sleeping bag with rain hammering on the tent and a cold wind swirling around outside, my thoughts turned to those friends and acquaintances I knew in the sailing world who had been lost at sea and who had never returned from their last voyage. Some had been lost whilst alone, some had left a shocked crew behind to endeavour to continue the voyage and bring their vessel home and some had gone down with the loss of the boat and all its crew. Many of these people were household names who had achieved great success on the oceans of the world, others were merely doing what they liked best – sailing a small boat without fuss across the world's oceans.

Soon after that trip to North Wales I decided to write about some of the sailors who I had known and who had been lost at sea. Some had been good friends. Others I had met in passing or whilst taking part in races or regattas.

I have been sailing all my life and in 1977 I first got involved in the world of fast racing multihulls. I took part in the 1978 Two Handed Round Britain and Ireland Race on a 35-foot trimaran, where I first met several of the people who feature in this book. Rob James was sailing with Chay Blyth in the monstrous trimaran *Great Britain IV* (which I later campaigned for a season) and I renewed a childhood friendship with Philip Walwyn who raced in his trimaran *Whisky Jack*, which he sold to me after the race.

Two years before that another friend, Mike McMullen, had been lost in his trimaran *Three Cheers* whilst taking part in the 1976 Observer Single-Handed Transatlantic Race, the OSTAR. The next year, 1977, the famous mountaineer / explorer / sailor Bill Tilman, with whom I had nearly sailed to Greenland in my university 'gap' year, was lost in the South Atlantic. He was on board the converted tug *En Avant* which disappeared, along with its entire crew, on passage to the Falkland Islands. Tilman was celebrating his 80th birthday by sailing to the South Atlantic on an expedition aiming to climb a mountain on Smith Island.

In 1979 I was the last person to see off the trimaran *Bucks Fizz* as it set sail to take part in that year's ill-fated Fastnet Race. *Bucks Fizz*, a near sister ship to the famous *Three Cheers*, was owned and sailed by another friend, Richard Pendred, and he and his crew were amongst the many fatalities of that race.

The next year, 1980, the British yacht designer Angus Primrose and his boat *Demon of Hamble* were lost off the South East coast of the USA. A year before, I had had discussions with him about the possibility of my building a yacht to one of his designs.

Over the years I have sailed to France to take part in several of their multihull races and regattas, most noticeably the 'Trophee des Multicoques' held annually at La Trinité-sur-Mer in Brittany. There I met many of the illustrious Frenchmen who had developed this sport and who had achieved near 'rock star' status in their own country. Amongst these were Alain Colas, who was lost at sea on board his world girdling trimaran *Manureva* whilst taking part in one of the Route de Rhum single handed races and Eric Tabarly, the most famous of them all, who fell overboard from his beloved yacht *Pen Duick* in 1998 and was lost whilst sailing up the Irish Sea on passage to Scotland.

I also write about the double tragedy of Peter Tangvald, a Norwegian yachtsman whom I first met in 1959, and his son Thomas. Peter spent his whole life wandering the world's oceans and was lost when his yacht hit a reef in the Caribbean in 1991. In 2014 his son, Thomas, was also lost at sea whilst alone on passage from French Guiana to Brazil.

I start the book with a description of the tragic first and last voyage, in 1949, of Frank and Ann Davison in their yacht *Reliance*, during which Frank was lost and the boat wrecked. Ann was a friend of an old aunt of mine who, many years ago now, told me about these events.

I also recount the strange last voyage of Donald Crowhurst in his trimaran *Teignmouth Electron*. He wandered the waters of the South Atlantic whilst pretending he was hurtling around the world via Cape Horn in pursuit of the Golden Globe Trophy for the first person to sail alone around the world non-stop. A film of this story, *The Mercy*, staring Colin Firth was released the day this book was published.

I end the book by describing the extraordinary life of an old childhood friend, Philip Walwyn, who tragically lost his life in 2015 only 10 miles from his destination at the end of a solo transatlantic voyage on his 12 Metre yacht *Kate*.

For obvious reasons there are few accounts of such last voyages. Often there have been no survivors to tell the story and such accounts as do exist are often mere conjecture. Whilst nowadays few sea passages end in disaster there is a poignancy about those that do, especially when a sailor is alone on the high seas and is overwhelmed by accident or stress of bad weather. The wide ocean can be a very lonely place, as can the narrow sea when tragedy strikes close to land at the end of a long voyage.

Chapter 1

The Last Voyage of Ann and Frank Davison and the Loss of the *Reliance* (1949)

An ageing aunt of mine first told me about her friend Ann Davison and the tragic voyage of the *Reliance*, which led to the loss of Ann's husband Frank. When I was young this aunt was an exotic figure who lived alone in a mews house in South Kensington and worked at the Foreign Office. At the age of twenty, at the start of the Second World War, she had married an RAF bomber pilot. He was killed six weeks later. For the rest of the war she did something secret at Bletchley Park and later worked for, and became the lover of, Frank Birch, the head of Bletchley's Naval Section. He was one of the people who helped crack the Enigma code. After the war she helped Frank Birch write the official history of British Signals Intelligence during the war.

My aunt Monica was one of the first women in England to own her own sailing boat. Soon after the end of World War II, she bought a series of old gaff cutters which she kept on the Helford River in Cornwall, looked after by a local boatman. One of these yachts was an old Falmouth Quay Punt called *Curlew*, which later achieved fame in the hands of Tim and Pauline Carr. They spent many years on her cruising the world to far flung places including time spent on South Georgia in Antarctica. *Curlew* has now ended her sailing days and is exhibited at the

National Maritime Museum in Falmouth.

Monica escaped to Cornwall whenever she could get away from London. It was during one of these visits that she met Ann Davison who was preparing her boat to become the first woman to sail across the Atlantic alone in her small yacht *Felicity Ann*. When I was a schoolboy, Monica gave me a copy of the book Ann had written about her life with, and the death of, her husband Frank – a story which fascinated me ever after. The book, first published in 1950, was called *Last Voyage* and was subtitled 'An autobiographical account of all that led up to an illicit voyage and the outcome thereof'. Some years later Monica gave me a copy of Ann's next book, called *My Ship Is So Small*, describing her Atlantic trip.

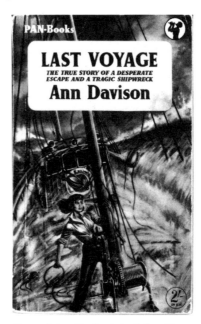

Cover of Ann Davison's book Last Voyage

Frank and Ann Davison were free spirits who first met in the years leading up to the Second World War. When he was young, Frank left England for Canada, worked as a lumberjack, panned for gold, gambled successfully on the grain market and then lost all his profits in a failing oil company. He raced motor cars and drove huskies across the Canadian snows. He sailed a small yacht single-handed back to England, where he taught himself to fly. In 1934, having got married, he took over a near derelict aerodrome on the Cheshire side of the River Mersey. There he built up a business offering charter flights, aerial photography and anything else that came along.

Ann had been born into a family of artists in England. She went to Veterinary College determined to 'do something with horses', became engaged to, and then ditched, a fellow. She became obsessed with aviation. In the 1930s she was one of the very first women in England to have qualified as a commercial pilot. She eked out a living working freelance doing charter flights, mail delivery by air around the UK and whatever else she could pick up.

In 1937 Frank advertised for a pilot to fly out of Blackpool, offering joy rides to holiday makers. Ann, who was seeking a change in her life, answered the advertisement and was taken on.

Ann shared Frank's love of variety, excitement and adventure. They had much in common and, after a while, fell in love. Frank divorced his first wife, Joy, in 1939 and that same year he and Ann were married. Sadly, Joy was killed in a flying accident the next year.

Their business prospered and Frank was full of ideas to expand further. He planned to build a make of Dutch aeroplane in the United Kingdom and hatched plans for an aerial bus route linking towns in the north west of England when the Second World War broke out.

Three days before the declaration of war the Air Ministry grounded all civilian aircraft. Then they requisitioned the aerodrome and the house in which Frank and Ann lived. The aircraft and everything else were bundled out of the hangers and stored in a nearby grandstand where the entire lot was destroyed by a fire, started by an intruder. No one in authority wanted anything to do with the situation and no proper compensation was ever agreed or paid. The RAF was not interested in Frank, he was considered too old, and nobody at that stage of the war wanted a female pilot.

So they moved on. Frank's family had an interest in some gravel quarries in Flintshire and Frank decided to develop one of these. A contract with the Air Ministry to supply gravel for a large project in Birkenhead was signed. A large mortgage was taken out to pay for it all.

Then, as so often in Frank's life, things began to fall apart. An exceptionally severe winter, with heavy frosts and snowfall, brought production to a halt. With no revenue coming in, mortgage payments were missed. When production started again Frank offered to pay off the arrears but the mortgage company refused these and promptly foreclosed on him.

This hit the two badly and Frank began to doubt his abilities, became bitter and withdrawn. Left with nothing but a small income from a smallholding run by Ann, they came across R M Lockley's books *Dream Island* and *Island Days*, telling of his life on the island of Skokholm off the Pembrokeshire coast.

Frank thought that Lockley had hit on something and said to Ann: "That's what I should like to do. Get to hell and gone from all this bloody turmoil and farm one of those little islands.... No bureaucratic busybodies, no ruddy argument. Not a goddam' soul. Bliss." So they started to look for an island.

This was not something easy to come by in the middle of a war but eventually they did find one, Inchmurrin, on Loch Lomond. They took on a tenancy, moved in, chartered a 4 ½ ton sloop in which Ann learned to sail and started a new life. They spent ten months on the island and it nearly broke their hearts. Everything which could go wrong went wrong. The goats died from eating grass infected by parasites, the geese eggs did not hatch and Frank's bank foreclosed on a small mortgage left over from the quarry and grabbed everything in his account.

They surrendered their tenancy and moved to another island on the loch called Inchfad. This was a better proposition, despite having no electricity or plumbing. Water was drawn from the loch by bucket. They continued to raise goats and geese, which prospered, and Ann started writing and selling magazine articles. They bought an old lifeboat and an engine from the Ministry of Transport which they converted into a barge.

But, despite this relative success and being the types of people they were, they soon became restless again. Ann told Frank that she could do with some 'real gut-stirring' as she put it and Frank agreed. They talked of emigrating and travelling around the world but doing it slowly. One day in 1945, just after the war ended, Frank returned to the island from a business trip with a sheaf of papers – a list of yachts for sale.

By now they had developed their idea into a simple plan – get hold of a boat and take it on a slow trip around the world, stopping at the first place they came to which they liked enough in which to settle. They reckoned they needed £2,000 for a boat and £1,000 in cash. If they could sell the island they would go, if they couldn't they would stay.

In 1946 they did find a buyer and sold the island and their livestock for a good price. They kept only their Alsatian dog and two goats, which they proposed to take with them on their boat (if it was large enough). Ann had persuaded Frank that this was not a crazy idea and reminded him that sailors used to take goats on sailing ships for a milk supply.

Ann and Frank left the island, boarded their animals with friends and started a search for a ship: a hard thing to do at that time. Most private yachts had been laid up during the war or had been requisitioned by the Navy. Others had had their lead or iron keels and other metal work removed to help the war effort. The search took them from Fort William in Scotland to the South Coast of England, to Bristol, Swansea and Ireland. They looked at a 50-foot MFV offered at £400, a Bristol Channel pilot cutter, a rusting steel schooner, a Brixham trawler, a pretty Swedish-built yawl and a Baltic trading schooner. Finally, they found a heavily-built fishing boat berthed in Fleetwood in Lancashire, named *Reliance*. She had been built in Fleetwood in 1903 on the lines of a yacht and named after the winner of that year's America's Cup.

Frank appointed Humphrey Barton, a yacht surveyor working in Jack Laurent Giles' office in Lymington, to survey *Reliance*. After giving her a good going over, Barton said he thought she was sound and that Frank might make something of her. They bought her for £1,450. What they got was just a hull, a rusty engine, some bits of equipment and some old sails, but little more.

By today's standards the *Reliance* was huge, 70 feet long with a beam of 18 feet and a draught of 9 feet 6 inches. She was massively built of pitch pine on oak and had once been rigged as a gaff ketch. On deck she was a grim mess with old worn out gear everywhere. Below decks she was even worse and in the engine room there was an old rusting Gardner 26VT two-cylinder diesel with compressed air starting which had been installed in 1925.

Frank and Ann moved to Fleetwood to start fitting out the old boat. At first they lived ashore then moved on board to save money. The original plan was simple: re-step and re-rig the masts, have new sails made, renew some decking and strengthen the wheelhouse. But, as anyone who has taken on the renovation of an old yacht knows only too well, things seldom work out like that.

Not only was Frank a perfectionist but, as so often happens, he became too enamoured with the boat: the amount of work expanded and everything had to be carried out to the highest quality. They started on a complete renovation of the interior. Later it was found that the engine had to be virtually rebuilt and the massive wooden bearers supporting the engine renewed. Shipwrights and engineers were engaged, sails and materials ordered. The vessel, moored alongside the town quay in full public view, became the talk of the town with much muttering from the local fishing community that maybe the new owners had taken on too much. Against this, her quality of build and her sailing abilities were well known and approved of.

Soon problems began to pile up one on top of another. Materials were hard, and sometimes impossible, to come by, costs escalated and the engine, once rebuilt, was almost impossible to start. (It took at least two people and some two hours to achieve this. First a compressor on a generator had to be run to pressurise a large air bottle. Then a blow lamp had to be aimed at the two cylinder heads to heat them until virtually red hot. When all was ready, the fly wheel had to be levered by hand with a crow bar until correctly aligned. Then a valve was opened and the engine might start. If not, the whole process had to be gone through again.)

Much of the work turned out to have been poorly done but full payment was still demanded. Debts began to mount and money began to run out. Their best shipwright deserted them and the Davison's were forced to consider taking paying crew with them for their voyage. They tried to arrange a charter and Frank nearly pulled off a job to act as base ship for a diving film to be shot in the Pacific. Soon invoices went unpaid and writs began to fly. Ann raised some money from writing articles and from the sales of a book she wrote about their island life but this was not enough.

Then a man from the Ministry of Shipping visited them and asked searching questions of their plans. After this Frank became convinced they were being watched by local Customs officers and he was sure he saw strange men hanging around the quay from time to time. They hatched plans as to how they were to get their money out of the country. At that time the amount allowed was limited to £50 per person.

In the summer of 1948, suddenly and out of the blue, their bank demanded full repayment of its loan. They knew this could end everything but they managed to persuade the bank to give them six months to sell *Reliance*. No buyer came forward and on Christmas Eve Frank and Ann received formal Notice of Foreclosure from the bank.

Matters dragged on over the next few months and in April

they learnt that *Reliance* had been placed in the hands of a ship-broker for auction. Then some people from whom Frank had borrowed £250 bought a summons against him. They had no money with which to pay and Frank and Ann knew that this was the end. They would lose a court case which would mean a writ nailed to the mast and ruination.

They played for time and got an adjournment of the summons until 17 May. Then one morning with only two weeks to go, Frank stopped what he was doing and said to Ann: "I can't stand any more of this. Let's clear out.... From now on the game is going to be played my way. To my rules. We will sail *Reliance* across to the States, or Cuba and we will have a chance to sell her for something like her value. It's our only chance of meeting these liabilities. And I'm damned if I am going to wait like a chicken for the axe."

"And we shall have had a sail," Ann said, in full agreement with Frank.

They knew they were leaving debts behind and that, once they set sail, it would be impossible to enter another port in the United Kingdom. But they were not prepared to give up their dream.

They made a plan to leave on Sunday 15 May, two days before the Court hearing and they started their preparations. To depart secretly was difficult as they still had to fuel and provision the ship. This they achieved with a great deal of subterfuge and with many silent night trips ashore. They managed to fob off officials from the Customs and the Ministry of Transport, the latter tipped off by the fuel company who provided the diesel Frank ordered. All the locals knew something was afoot.

On their chosen day they waited on board for the tide to rise sufficiently to float *Reliance*. They had put it about that they were only going out for engine trials. After one false start, when a vital piece of the engine broke and had to be replaced, delaying them some 48 hours, they slipped their mooring lines at high tide in the late afternoon of 17 May and motored out of the harbour.

As they motored down the channel past the fishing quays everyone stopped what they were doing and watched, in silence. No-one waved them off. The weather was dreadful and a lowering grey sky foretold strong winds to come. *Reliance* negotiated a dog leg in the harbour mouth and was soon out into the estuary heading for the Lune lightship. There they met a freshening south westerly wind. Unbeknownst to them, southerly gales were forecast.

With the sun setting, Frank turned *Reliance* onto a south westerly course so as to clear the Skerries off the coast of Anglesey. Now their real troubles and their nightmare voyage began. As the wind increased, large grey white capped rollers raced incessantly at them from ahead and, with no sail set, the old boat pitched and rolled ferociously. The first problem to emerge was with the sails. They were still unpacked in their original bags, lashed on deck. With a boat of that size it was impossible to bend the mainsail or mizzen onto the spars and set them in such conditions. The gaff and booms were enormous and little of the running rigging needed was in place. They did, however, manage to set an old staysail on the forestay and they hoisted the head of an old mizzen on the mainmast, as a sort of mainsail. This was done without a boom and the sail could not be made to set properly. Progress to windward under sail alone was impossible. This all took many hours and one of them had to go down to the engine room every few hours, day and night, to pump up fuel by hand into a small header tank which fed the engine.

Towards evening on the first day they spotted the Tuskar light on the Irish coast. Below decks all was chaos, but Ann was able to sort out a meal of sorts whilst Frank steered a course as best he could. They had never swung the compass, had no deviation card, and had no idea of their true heading. They saw nothing that night save the lights of a few fishing vessels.

Dawn brought a dreary sight of a heaving grey sea, an ever increasing wind and a low grey sky with frequent rain squalls and showers. Later they think they crossed the Nymph bank off the south of Ireland and ran into an ugly cross sea.

It is hard today to imagine just how alone they were at sea in those days. Whilst they had proper charts and pilot books (and Frank had and knew how to use a sextant) there were few, if any, navigation aids available to them. Weather forecasts were infrequent and mostly inaccurate. Buoyage was uncertain as were lights, there were no radio direction finding facilities then and they had no log to measure distance. All they had was an uncertain compass and some charts. Neither radio assistance nor shelter could be sought.

At one point during the second night the paraffin stove in the galley broke loose, spilled fuel over the floor and set the galley alight. Frank and Ann managed to put the fire out but it was a close run thing and left the galley and surrounding areas burnt and blistered and the crew very shaken.

For the next few days (here, in Ann's narrative, she became uncertain of how many days passed) *Reliance* headed steadily south and then, as the wind backed into the south, south east. They saw no land. At times they hove to and at other times ran with the wind, until they had lost all sense of direction. They

27

were hopelessly and completely lost. Frank now began to lose control after days standing at the wheel with no sleep. He began to hallucinate and rant and rage at Ann. Ann felt her own control slipping but valiantly tried to keep herself together whilst trying to keep Frank calm.

The wind never relented, the seas became larger and the sun never shone. Frank was not able to take a sun sight. One night they saw a light which Frank was convinced was the Skerries light off Anglesey but the flashes did not accord with the chart. Ann was convinced they were much further south.

Then the engine stopped. They left *Reliance* to look after herself whilst they tried to get it started. Eventually they succeeded. During another night, visibility cleared temporarily and they found themselves amongst breakers surrounded by flashing lights with rocks close by. Ann tried to work out from the charts where they might be but to no avail. Frank turned the boat round and tried to retrace their steps. At one point, *Reliance* struck the bottom with a sickening crash, keeled over alarmingly but slid off whatever they had hit. Soon they were back in deep water.

Then the engine stopped again. They continued under sail but could not make better than 90 degrees to the wind. By now they were both totally exhausted but they never thought of giving up. Frank said they would just have to beat out of the Channel as best they could and however long it took.

They began to see large ships and liners and slowly worked out that they were probably in the mouth of the English Channel. The best course they could set was a little east of south. They could only hope that the wind would eventually veer. At one point they saw land ahead, which they guessed was the French coast. They thought of trying to enter a French harbour for fuel and a rest but turned away.

They tacked back and forth across the Channel but were, in reality, making no progress and were being beaten remorselessly further and further east. One night, land and rocks appeared ahead of them. They had no engine and could not tack clear in time. They were forced to drop anchor in a small open rocky inlet. The anchor held but it was a lee shore with ugly looking rocks close astern. They were pitching badly and snatching savagely at the cable. The two went below and immediately fell into a deep sleep. Some hours later Ann was woken by voices and went on deck to find a fishing boat alongside, heaving up and down in the swell. The crew hailed them and said that the ship was in a dangerous situation and asked if they needed help. Frank appeared on deck, refused any such offer and said everything was fine. The fishermen repeated their offer and made off, shaking their heads. Why neither Frank nor Ann asked where they were will never be known.

The anchor would not hold for ever. The wind began to blow even harder and they knew they would never be able to sail out of the anchorage. They went below to see if the engine would start. After several hours they got it going and, with Ann at the wheel, Frank veered all the remaining anchor cable and let the bitter end run free. They resumed their battle and *Reliance* headed off once more to try to escape westwards and then southwards into warmer waters. Even with the engine going they could make little progress to windward.

They then had a short respite from the wind and one morning, after several tacks across the channel, they found themselves close to the Eddystone Lighthouse, off the entrance to Plymouth. A small fishing boat hailed them and asked if they needed help.

Frank also refused this offer, saying that they were just drying out after a bit of a pasting during the night. Frank hoisted a light weather jib and they spent the rest of that day slowly beating out into the Channel. By nightfall they were off the French coast, still hemmed in by the incessant westerly wind. They tacked back toward England and got trapped by wind and tide in Lyme Bay between Start Point and Portland Bill.

The wind started to blow up again and toward nightfall (Ann thought it was now 3 June) the jib burst and flogged itself to ribbons. They found themselves being drawn closer and closer to land and to Portland Bill. The lights behind Chesil Beach got brighter and brighter as did the lights on the tall radio masts on the Bill itself. They listened to a weather forecast predicting yet another gale from the south west. The tide was running at some six knots driving the boat inexorably towards the high cliffs off Portland. The engine was now firing on one cylinder only but half power was not enough.

Ann looked out of the wheelhouse door and saw black waves breaking on outlying rock pinnacles right in their path. Then finally the engine stopped and they knew they would never make it. They lit a paraffin soaked bundle of some of Ann's clothes as a flare. They were trying to put on life jackets when *Reliance* struck, lightly at first then harder and harder. Then the cliffs were upon them, the bowsprit snapped like a piece of kindling and the boat started to roll from side to side. The mast came crashing down and the bows buried into the cliff face. They threw a cork life float into the sea and Ann swung her legs over the side, fell into the float and clung on. Frank jumped into the sea and swam to the float. He cut the painter which tethered the float to the stricken yacht and they paddled clear. The cliffs were too steep to climb and they struck out along the coast in the direction of Weymouth. Their craft was a lozenge shaped ring of cork, covered in canvas with rope lifelines strung around it. In the middle was an empty wooden box in which they should have stored provisions and some water. As they paddled away from the wreck they saw activity on land. A rocket was fired and torches and car headlamps appeared. Obviously a rescue was in progress. All they had with them was a pocket knife and four £1 notes.

The current which had driven *Reliance* onto the rocks was now carrying the raft out to sea. Later that night a steamer passed close by but saw nothing. When the tide turned it carried the float back past the wreck and even further out to sea right into the centre of the infamous Portland Race. The seas got wilder and wilder with towering pinnacles of white water dashing into each other with bursts of foam. The float capsized again and again, throwing them into the water and they became weaker and weaker. On the top of one wave they saw Portland Bill in the distance, Frank stood up, looked and put out a hand to Ann, pressed hers and then smiled. Fading into unconsciousness he tried to climb out of the float. A monster wave rose above it and swept down upon them. Ann threw an arm around Frank but the sea tore him away and he was gone.

This was the last wave that broke on the float, which had now been driven free of the race and started to drift back to land. Ann passed a large brown buoy, which marked a sunken aircraft, twelve miles from land. As she neared land the float was driven at first toward a beach at the mainland end of the island then the tide turned and swept her seawards toward the Bill itself. Ann tried to paddle to steer the raft but was driven onto a mass of rocks and boulders at the very tip of the Bill. The float grounded, Ann climbed out and managed to climb the rocks until she came to a gentle slope leading to the radio masts and the lighthouse.

Frank's body was never found and little remained of *Reliance* amongst the rocks.

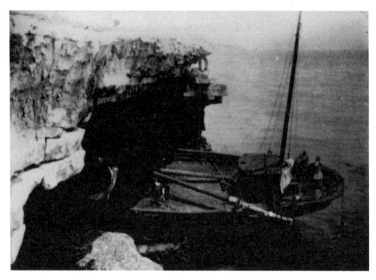

Reliance on the day after grounding on Portland Bill

I have often tried to work out from Ann's narrative the course *Reliance* actually took, but without much success. I think the first light they saw was off the Pembrokeshire coast, perhaps the Bishops or the Smalls. The ring of lights and rocks must have been off Land's End and they probably anchored somewhere near Mullion or off the Lizard. (According to one account, it was the Newlyn Lifeboat, and not a fishing boat, which came alongside when they were anchored. This would confirm the position of the anchorage as being on the west side of the Lizard.)

Soon after the tragedy, Ann got a job in a boatyard in the West Country and then tried to find a berth as crew. She wrote the account of the voyage of *Reliance* and, with the money she made from this, paid off all Frank's debts. In 1952 she bought herself a small yacht, the *Felicity Ann*, which she sailed to America. She was the first woman to sail solo across the Atlantic. Ann later remarried in America and died in 1992. She had no children.

Chapter 2

The Strange Last Voyage of Donald Crowhurst and the Trimaran *Teignmouth Electron* (1969)

The story of Donald Crowhurst's voyage in the trimaran *Teignmouth Electron* and its tragic ending is almost too well known to bear repeating. It has been the subject of a number of books, most notably that by Nicholas Tomalin and Ron Hall entitled *The Strange Voyage of Donald Crowhurst* and the subject of several films, including, most recently, *The Mercy*.

But it is worth looking again at some of the circumstances which led up to the voyage and as to when and why Crowhurst first decided to deceive the world of his actual plight. It will never be known whether his death was an accident or intentional. Whatever it was, he died in intolerable circumstances. The final stages of the voyage have a tragic inevitability about them which are truly awful. All could have been avoided or foreseen at a much earlier stage, had not those involved been swept up in Crowhurst's dreams of fame and glory.

*

In 1967 I bought my first sailing yacht, a small 22-foot gaff cutter which had been built on the River Exe in 1907 as a salmon fishing boat. She was called *Roma* and had been converted into a yacht in the 1920s. I found her in a mud berth in Cowes on the Isle of Wight, just returned from a trip to Morocco and sporting an African fence post as a temporary bowsprit.

The boat lacked any navigation equipment and in 1968 I looked around at the London Boat Show to see what cheap equipment was available. I was then very inexperienced (and poor) and knew little about how to navigate. At the Boat Show I came across a stand selling a piece of equipment which interested me. It was called a Navicator and was made by a company called Electron Utilisation based in the West Country. It was a radio direction finding device which seemed well designed and reasonably priced. The salesman was very enthusiastic and persuasive so I bought one there and then and took it home to try it out.

I can't remember now the reason why, but a few months later I telephoned the company to ask about some query I had. I spoke to a Mr Crowhurst who said he was the owner of the business. I recognised the upper class tones and somewhat high pitched nasal voice as that of the man who had sold me the instrument at the Boat Show. I was surprised to learn he was the boss and owner of the business. He was very helpful, took time to explain to me exactly how to use the instrument and asked me to keep in touch and to let him know how I got on at sea with it. I used it for many years but never contacted the company again. Radio direction finding is no longer in use but I probably still have the Navicator gathering dust somewhere amongst the large pile of old boat bits in my barn.

Naturally, therefore, I was interested when, the next year, I read that Donald Crowhurst had announced his intention to take part in the Sunday Times Golden Globe Single-Handed Non-

Stop Round the World Race. Crowhurst made his announcement four days after the Sunday Times first published the rules.

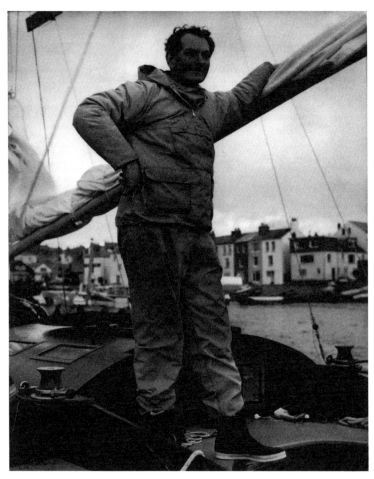

Donald Crowhurst on board Teignmouth Electron

What is less well known is that, for many months prior to this, Crowhurst had been trying to persuade Greenwich Council and

Donald Crowhurst, Teignmouth Electron (1969)

the Cutty Sark Society to lend him, for one year, Sir Francis Chichester's yacht *Gipsy Moth IV*. This was the yacht which had bought fame and fortune to Sir Francis following his solo round the world trip, at the end of which he was knighted by the Queen. Crowhurst put forward a proposal that he would sail the boat around the world non-stop and become the first man to achieve this. In return, he would hand over to the Council and the Society the large amount of money he would undoubtedly make from the voyage. He even agreed to make an immediate £5,000 donation and would hand over all the prize money he would win.

At that time, and to many people's alarm, *Gypsy Moth IV* was about to be sunk into concrete, seemingly for ever, in a specially built dry dock next to the *Cutty Sark* in Greenwich. Crowhurst's plan was refused but he did not give up. At the 1968 London Boat Show he lobbied various influential figures, including Angus Primrose (see Chapter 7), the designer of *Gipsy Moth IV*. Various yachting journals took up the cause opining strongly that boats, even famous ones, were meant to sail not sit in concrete. Sir Francis was approached to give his view about Crowhurst's proposal but was suspicious of him as he did not seem to be able to give any evidence of his competence. Chichester's scepticism played an increasing part in the Crowhurst story.

Nothing came of the plan and the boat was embedded in concrete where she sat disintegrating until 2013 when she was dug out, rebuilt and sailed around the world again (as described in the book *Gipsy Moth IV: The Legend Sails Again*). It is hard to imagine what would have happened had Crowhurst's wish been granted.

It is interesting to note that Crowhurst scoffed at all the fuss made at the time about Chichester's voyage, maintaining that Chichester had not achieved anything which had not already been done. On the day of Chichester's arrival in Plymouth, unlike most sailors who formed a huge armada to welcome their hero into harbour, Crowhurst instead spent the day sailing his boat alone off the north coast of Devon, away from all the fuss.

During all this lobbying, Crowhurst maintained that *Gipsy Moth IV* was the most suitable boat in existence for the voyage. As soon as his plan was rejected Crowhurst set about finding the money to build a boat of his own. This time, the type of boat he wanted could not have been more different. He had suddenly become converted to the benefits of multihulls and trimarans in particular (and this even without his ever having sailed one).

It was now May of 1968 and, in order to take part in the race, Crowhurst had to have a boat ready to set off by the end of October, the last date on which a competitor could leave. Hardly enough time for anyone to design, build, fit out, work up and equip a boat for a solo non-stop round the world trip, which most people thought was impossible anyway. But, undaunted, this was just the sort of challenge which Crowhurst relished.

Despite the grand old man's criticisms of his own boat (most of which, as we shall see later in this book, were self-serving or brought about as a result of the designer being forced to incorporate Chichester's own ideas), Crowhurst was probably right when he said *Gipsy Moth IV* was the best boat in which he could conquer 'the Everest of the Sea' as he described the venture. But at that time, a new monohull like Chichester's would have been far too expensive and would have taken far too long to build. Anyhow, Crowhurst did not have any money. Glass reinforced plastic boats were then in their infancy and Crowhurst had little option other than to find a stock boat that he could adapt to his purposes. And a cheap one.

Crowhurst's decision to go for a trimaran was actually far sighted and undoubtedly the right one, even though multihull development was in its infancy and despite the fact that Crowhurst had never sailed one. In the early sixties Arthur Piver, an American airline pilot and yacht designer, was the first person to popularise the building of trimarans by producing designs which could easily and cheaply be built by amateurs. Piver himself perished at sea in March 1968 while sailing one of his own designs, the presumed victim of a multihull's one major drawback – their inability to right themselves after a capsize.

Crowhurst was probably more influenced by Derek Kelsall, the British yacht designer who, in 1964, sailed a Piver trimaran, *Folatre*, in the second Observer Singlehanded Transatlantic Race (always known as the OSTAR). Two years later Kelsall won the first Round Britain and Ireland Race in his own designed and built trimaran, *Toria*. She was staggeringly fast for her day, completing the 2,000-mile course in eleven sailing days. *Toria* was very different from the narrow beamed 'v' shaped hulls of the Piver boats, and was the way forward for all future multihull development.

Crowhurst next set about finding a source of money to build his dream boat. He persuaded a West Country business man, Stanley Best, to be his source. Crowhurst asked him for £6,000 but this soon had to be doubled to £12,000. Crowhurst described multihulls as 'caravans of the sea', which no doubt appealed to caravan site owner Stanley Best, who had earlier put money into Crowhurst's company Electron Utilisation. Terms were agreed but there was one clause in Best's agreement which weighed deeply on Crowhurst's mind throughout his voyage and which contributed to its tragic ending. Best stipulated that, if anything went wrong with the voyage, he, Best, would have the option to sell the boat back to Electron Utilisation: something for which Crowhurst did not have the money. Thus, if the voyage failed, Crowhurst would be ruined. (Best later said he only inserted this clause for tax reasons and never intended that it should be implemented.)

Crowhurst now had to find a boatyard that could build his trimaran cheaply and in time for the end of October deadline. With the deadline five months away, Crowhurst settled on two things, first he would buy the three hulls of a standard 41-foot trimaran of the Piver 'Victress' design, which were being built on a production line basis by Cox Marine in Essex. He would then get the trimaran put together by a small boatyard on the Norfolk Broads, who had promised they could finish it by the end of August and at a reasonable price.

At about this time Crowhurst learnt that another person was also intending to join the race in a Victress trimaran, a naval commander called Nigel Tetley. His boat was called *Victress*. This gave Crowhurst an added spur to make his boat leaner, lighter and faster than Tetley's which was fitted out as the family's floating home (most definitely a caravan of the sea). Tetley's *Victress* was built as a cruising boat, pure and simple, designed for comfort with a large living space and for upright sailing. She was rigged as a ketch, with a boomed self-tacking staysail; an ideal cruising rig but not what one would choose for a racing yacht. In many ways, she was one of the most unsuitable boats you could think of for an epic round the world non-stop single handed race, but she was all Tetley had and she would have to do.

The three hulls for Crowhurst's boat were delivered to Norfolk on 28 July as promised, giving the boatyard, Eastwoods (who had never built a trimaran before), the almost impossible task of completing the job in time. Crowhurst decided to have the boat flush decked with only a small cockpit and doghouse. This was a sensible idea in view of the seas in which he would be sailing, but it also meant that the trimaran would be cheaper and quicker to build. He also proposed a revolutionary system to prevent a capsize: a real possibility with all multihulls. His system was to have electrodes built in the side of the hulls which would send signals to what Crowhurst termed his 'computer' which would then fire off a carbon dioxide cylinder connected to a buoyancy bag strapped to the top of the mast. This would prevent a complete inversion and water would then be pumped into the upper hull which would eventually flip the boat upright. All this was to be controlled by his computer. Crowhurst announced to the world that his system had been tested, was fully operational and was the result of development by his company, Electron Utilisation.

Unfortunately, this was all total nonsense and when Crowhurst departed on his voyage none of the wires and pipes the builders had installed were connected up or went anywhere. There never was any such thing as his 'computer'.

Whatever may be said about Crowhurst, he had an extraordinary talent for making people believe him. He had impressed all his friends, impressed the yacht designer Angus Primrose, convinced a pragmatic Stanley Best and impressed John Eastwood, the builder of the boat. Even the Sunday Times reported that he was an experienced sailor. His only actual sailing experience was coast hopping along the Devon coast line.

Now all he had to do was to find a sponsor to publicise his

voyage and raise some funds. By chance the Sunday Times commissioned a small local news agency to photograph the unknown entrant in the race. This was the Devon News Agency, owned by Rodney Hallworth, who immediately spotted an opportunity and who came to play a large part in the upcoming tragedy. Hallworth told Crowhurst that, if he agreed to start the race from Teignmouth and used the town's name, he would find sponsors and get him all the money and publicity he would want. Crowhurst agreed and suggested Electron of Teignmouth for the name. "No," said Hallworth, "it must be *Teignmouth Electron*." Hallworth set to work but was woefully unsuccessful in raising money.

Meanwhile in Norfolk, the launch day came and went. A new date of 12 September was fixed and things began to go even more wrong. On 21 September (two days before the next agreed launch date) Crowhurst and Eastwoods had an angry discussion when Crowhurst was told that there was no time for the decks of the boat to be sheathed in fibreglass (which was part of the boat's specification and essential for preserving its structural integrity). Eastwoods said that they would merely be painted. It was too late in the day to do anything but agree. Crowhurst's wife pleaded with Donald to refuse delivery of the boat and abandon the project. Crowhurst replied that he had to go through with it adding "I'll just have to build the boat myself on the way round."

Teignmouth Electron was eventually launched into the River Yare on 23 September and following furious arguments with Eastwoods about money and how to rig the boat, she was pronounced ready to sail on 2 October. Crowhurst set out from Great Yarmouth with two friends at two o'clock in the morning of the next day to sail the boat to Teignmouth. They aimed to make the trip in three days. It actually took them 13 (at an average speed of only 23 miles per day), leaving them 16 days to get ready for the start, a virtually impossible task. On the trip they found the boat difficult to balance, the sails did not set properly and they could hardly get her to sail to windward at all. None of the hatches on the floats fitted properly and the floats filled with water. The self-steering gear was designed for monohulls and could not cope with the acceleration and the vibration set up by the faster moving multihull – the screws in the gear shook themselves loose every few hours.

One night on this trip Peter Beard, a good friend of Crowhurst and an experienced sailor, queried how on earth Crowhurst was going to get his boat round the world. Donald's response was that the winds would be favourable and mostly from behind. Beard asked what would happen if they weren't. Crowhurst is reputed to have replied that one could always meander around in the South Atlantic for a few months. He then drew a rough map circling an area off South America remarking that there were empty places out there where no one would ever find a small boat like his.

If this is true, then it means that Crowhurst must have had his plan to deceive everyone very much in mind from the start.

The next sixteen days in Teignmouth were chaos. The boat was lifted out of the water for repairs and for extensive leaks to be fixed. Piles of equipment arrived to be stored on board. Crowhurst went around in a daze. A BBC crew arrived to film the preparations and, sensing a tragedy not a triumph, changed the tone of their filming. A trial sail showed up more weaknesses and important fittings pulled out from the deck. The day before departure the boat was far from ready and the BBC crew gave

43

up filming to help with the preparations. That evening there was a dinner for Crowhurst's family and friends, at which the mood was described as funereal.

Later that night Donald confessed to his wife, Clare, that the boat was not ready and was not right. He asked her whether she would go out of her mind with worry if he left with the boat in this awful state. She replied by asking him, if he gave up now, would he be unhappy for the rest of his life? Crowhurst did not answer but started to cry. He wept for the rest of the night.

The weather on 31 October was miserable. At three o'clock in the afternoon, with only hours to go to the deadline, *Teignmouth Electron* was towed out to sea. Things immediately began to go wrong. The sail halyards had been rigged incorrectly and were trapped by the inflation device at the masthead. Much to the delight of some watching sceptics, the boat was towed back to harbour. The mess was sorted and the boat was towed out to sea again. A few minutes before five o'clock, a gun was fired and *Teignmouth Electron* crossed the start line.

*

Before considering Crowhurst's voyage it is worth digressing here to try to understand just what it was that made *Teignmouth Electron* such a poor performer and what made her so unsuitable for the venture she was about to undertake. Quite apart from the fact that the boat was quite unready, she should really never have left Teignmouth and she never stood a chance of completing the intended voyage. The boat was fundamentally flawed and no one seemed to have addressed the problems at the time. It was a classic case of 'the emperor's new clothes' and no one stood up and said "STOP".

No proper thought went into how to rig *Teignmouth Electron* and this was another sign of Crowhurst's inexperience. Despite his being meant to organise the rig and sails himself, he became immersed in his 'electronics' and left it entirely to Eastwoods to design the rig. Eastwoods had no multihull experience and simply adopted a standard Victress rig but with a shorter and heavier main mast, 38-foot instead of 42-foot (this was necessary because of the extra stresses and strains imposed on the mast from Crowhurst's self-righting system). The sails Eastwoods ordered were cut too full for a multihull, fouled the rigging and could not be set properly.

In addition to this *Teignmouth Electron* was built lighter than a standard Victress trimaran and the decks, which form part of the main structure holding the floats together, were not sheathed in fibreglass as specified. This would have led to a very flexible structure which would inevitably start to break up, as it did. Further, the heavier masts on *Teignmouth Electron* would have exacerbated another problem inherent in all multihulls – persistent pitching in a seaway. This not only reduces speed but puts additional strain on the structure and on the rig.

No wonder therefore that it took them thirteen days and not three to sail from Norfolk to Teignmouth and that it was almost impossible to get the boat to go to windward. Why, on arrival at Teignmouth, did nobody say or do anything about the rig and sails or call in an expert to give some advice? Crowhurst could even have called on one of his admirers – Angus Primrose (see Chapter 7). In fact, the whole vessel was put together on the back of an envelope, without any professional or expert opinion whatsoever.

It is a sign of Crowhurst's ignorance (or arrogance) that he never seems to have seriously considered this problem. More thought was given to his 'electronics' than to how to power the vessel to make it sail properly and faster.

So the fact is that, however good a sailor Crowhurst might have been, and, however hard or expertly Crowhurst might have sailed his boat, he would never have been able to achieve his ambition or the speeds he was forecasting. The venture was doomed from the outset.

*

I will not describe his trip in detail. It has all been done before and Crowhurst's log books describe an all too painful account of a growing awareness by him that he could never achieve what he had set out to do.

After 2 weeks at sea he set out in his log book the pros and cons of going on or giving up. He must, by then, have become aware that no-one in his right senses would take such a vessel into the Roaring Forties. He prevaricated but decided to carry on whilst trying to get his generator working so that he could talk to Stanley Best on the radio. He made two versions of a written assessment of his predicament: one on heroic lines for public consumption and a real one which was a realistic summing up of his situation and it set out all the reasons why he could not take his boat into the Southern Ocean. The self-steering could not stop the boat from broaching; there was no way to pump out the leaking floats other than opening up the leaking hatches and bailing with a bucket – suicide in the bad seas to be expected further south; his electrics and chronometer had given up and he had no way of getting time signals; the sails were all cut wrongly and too full (at last an acknowledgement that there was some-thing wrong with the rig); there was no way of pumping out the main hull; the cockpit hatch leaked onto the generator. The list went on and on.

He eventually got the generator working and, in mid-Novem-ber, spoke to Clare, his wife, and to Stanley Best. In his log he had written that he would raise all these problems and ask for advice as to whether he should give up. However, all he did was merely discuss minor problems and he never raised the possibil-ity of giving up. He did the same when he talked again to Best a few days later. He completely avoided discussing the main issue: should he continue?

He was making steady but slow progress down the Atlantic and he passed the Canary Islands at the end of November. After that it is hard to establish just where he was or what his intentions were. Sometime around mid-December he started to invent his position and he began to send cables which were ambiguous in the extreme as to his real position; almost anything could be read into their wording. Hallworth, of course, interpreted them in the best possible light, adding to the confusion.

From then on his fake position got further and further from his real position. As he did this, things got more and more difficult. Before the days of electronic calculators or computers, faking a position and making an astronomical calculation backwards from an imaginary position to get a sextant angle at an exact time of day is a very difficult, almost impossible, thing to do and requires many complicated mathematical calculations. He also had to invent weather reports and describe sailing conditions he never encountered, all things which must be in a log book which he knew would be subject to inspection on his return. Especially if he won.

Interestingly, Crowhurst was not the only competitor who toyed with this idea. When things were very difficult for him, John Ridgeway, another competitor in the race, admitted considering simply resting in the sun for a year and then returning saying he had been all the way round. But he quickly discounted this as he did not believe he could carry it off or live with himself afterwards.

In January Crowhurst cabled that, anticipating bad weather in the Southern Ocean, he was sealing the hatch in the cockpit floor over his generator and that radio messages would become much less frequent. He had to do this as he could not send messages to Australia or New Zealand whilst still in the South Atlantic – he had to wait for his false position to catch up with his true position on his real way home. His position now given to the press was over 4,000 miles away from his true position.

Whilst apparently hurtling across the Southern Ocean, Crowhurst was actually limping toward the coast of South America, with a very damaged boat. The plywood skin of one of his hulls had split and the hull was leaking badly. He needed to put into port to make repairs.

Now begins the most extraordinary event of his whole 'non-stop' voyage. Could Crowhurst find somewhere where he could land unnoticed and unreported and find materials for the repair? He studied his pilot books and decided to make for land 600 miles south of the entrance to the River Plate and Buenos Aires. When approaching land, he closed with the wide bay of Bahia Samborombon. Here the pilot book said there was an anchorage off the River Salado, where there was a small settlement.

Crowhurst arrived and dropped anchor on 6 March 1969. He had been at sea for just over five months.

Crowhurst anchored right under the noses of the local Coastguard station, charged with observing shipping entering and leaving the River Plate. His name was entered in the station's log simply as Charles Alfred, these being Crowhurst's two middle names. The Coastguard said that they had to contact the authorities in Buenos Aries for instructions and this got Crowhurst very agitated. Unbelievably, the Coastguard had no telephone and someone was sent off to find the nearest one and deliver the message. Luckily for Crowhurst, the message never got through.

Despite language difficulties, and whilst waiting to be discovered, Crowhurst managed to get across that he was in a sailing race, had rounded Cape Horn, was on his way home to England and he needed materials to repair his boat. He spent the night on board, was given the materials he needed and the next morning set about the repairs, which took two days. On the morning of the third day, still with no word from the authorities, he was towed out to sea and he left.

During the rest of March, Crowhurst dawdled around and wandered towards the Falkland Islands. He worked at his false log book. He calculated that at a notional 140 miles a day he could pretend to round Cape Horn on 15 April. He approached close to the Falkland Islands, possibly to get a taste of South Atlantic weather and possibly to photograph land. He then set off toward home and in early April sent a cryptic message saying he was nearing Cape Horn.

Hallworth was ecstatic and replied informing Crowhurst that he was not far behind Tetley and suggested a photo finish would make great news. He also said that Knox-Johnston (who had started earlier) was expected home in one or two weeks.

Crowhurst continued to meander up the South Atlantic until 4 May when his fictional position eventually met up with where he really was. On 30 April, a few days before this, he broke radio silence with another cryptic message declaring himself back in the race.

With Robin Knox-Johnston heading north on the last stretch of the Atlantic and on course to win the Golden Globe award (for first home), he, Crowhurst, and the only remaining competitor, Nigel Tetley in his trimaran *Victress*, were now left to battle it out for the £5,000 prize for the fastest voyage. At first Crowhurst put on a 'real' spurt and sent cables announcing his progress. Hallworth replied with glowing cables telling Crowhurst of the welcome which was waiting for him.

Suddenly Crowhurst slowed down and sent cables emphasising problems with the boat. Had Crowhurst hit on one last way out − to lose the race. If he lost to Tetley he would lose the £5,000 but he could arrive quietly in second place. No one would examine his log books. He could still claim a successful voyage and Stanley Best would not be able to invoke his option to require him to buy the boat.

Around this time Crowhurst learnt that a second possible escape route had also disappeared. The Frenchman Bernard Moitessier, another competitor in his steel ketch *Joshua*, had been coming up the Atlantic fast behind Knox-Johnston and might have overtaken him and put up the fastest time to win both trophies (allowing Crowhurst to slow down and come in second or third). But Moitessier suddenly declared that he was resigning from the race. He peeled off to the right, sailed round the Cape of Good Hope for a second time, sailed across the Indian Ocean and south of Australia and New Zealand again. He then sailed off into the wide open spaces of the tropical Pacific Ocean, 'to save my soul' as he put it. He almost sailed twice round the world without stopping.

Tetley, thinking Crowhurst was coming up fast behind him, pushed on harder than ever. *Victress* was falling apart but Tetley, aware that 'his' prize was about to be taken from his grasp, was determined to keep afloat and get his boat to England come what may. But the trimaran could not take it and began to break up. He staggered on but ran into a gale when near the Azores and, just after midnight on 21 May, his port float broke off, smashed into the centre hull and *Victress* began to sink. He took to a life raft. He was 1,200 miles from home and had already crossed his outward path. *Victress* had become the first trimaran to circumnavigate the world and would, in all likelihood, have made it home had Tetley not pushed her so hard in his attempt to keep ahead of his apparent rival. The next day he was picked up by an Italian oil tanker.

The irony of this was exquisite. Crowhurst, through his deceit, now faced the biggest dilemma of his life. What was he to do? If he returned home, he could not but avoid winning with all that that entailed. His lies had not only sunk Tetley but also his own last chance to escape.

For the next few weeks Crowhurst continued to sail northward and appeared to be acting normally but, to anyone reading his logs, it is clear that his mind was deeply disturbed. The mental stresses and strains on him were by now intolerable. He sent out cables to his wife and to others in which he appeared rational and sane when he was, in reality, far from it. He was now in the Sargasso Sea and he gave up sailing completely, allowing the boat to look after herself. He withdrew into himself and began to write in a new log book. He covered page after page in incoherent thoughts about God, the cosmic mind, game playing with God, mathematics, Einstein and relativity, man becoming God and leaving the physical world behind. At the same time, he became desperate to talk to his wife and spent hour after hour trying to repair his radio transmitter. The repair failed and Crowhurst went completely to pieces and descended into madness.

Crowhurst had become convinced that, at a future self-appointed time, he could leave his physical body and enter another dimension of abstract existence. The rest is speculation but Nicholas Tomalin and Ron Hall, in their book about the voyage, presume that Crowhurst took the boat's chronometer off the cabin bulkhead (it was missing) and walked with it to the stern of the boat and then, at the exact time he had stated in his log that he would 'resign the game', jumped off the stern into the sea.

On 10 July the Royal Mail vessel *Picardy* spotted a yacht drifting with only its mizzen sail up. No one was on deck. The ship closed with the yacht and saw it was a trimaran called *Teignmouth Electron*. They sounded their foghorn. No one appeared. They lowered a boat to investigate and found the yacht abandoned.

They were in the middle of the Atlantic half way between Europe and the Caribbean. They hoisted the trimaran onto the deck of the ship and proceeded toward Jamaica. The ship's captain read Crowhurst's logs and writings and sent a cable to London. This was when the world first learned of what had happened.

The trimaran was off-loaded in Jamaica and later sold off at auction. The new owner took her to Grand Cayman Island where, in due course, she was damaged in a hurricane. She was beached on Cayman Brac where she remains to this day, lying near the shore, a broken decaying hulk dead and forgotten. There she will surely end her days.

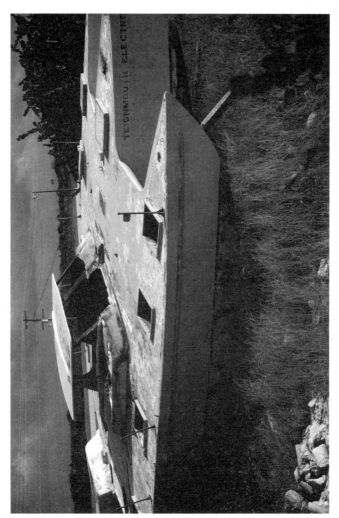

Donald Crowhurst's Teignmouth Electron on Cayman Brac, Cayman Islands in 1991

Chapter 3

The Life and Last Voyage of Mike McMullen and the Trimaran *Three Cheers* (1976)

Two virtual sister ships were involved in two tragic voyages under entirely separate circumstances, unrelated to each other or to any defects in their design or build. One voyage on the trimaran *Three Cheers* was made in 1976 and the other on the trimaran *Bucks Fizz* took place during the fateful Fastnet Race of 1979 (see Chapter 6).

*

In the late 1960s Dick Newick was a visionary yacht designer working out of St Croix in the US Virgin Islands in the Caribbean, beginning to make a name for himself in the then emerging world of multihulls. He began to produce a series of sleek, contoured and very fast two and three hulled yachts. They looked different from anything that had come before and took their inspiration from ancient Polynesian outrigger canoes. They were fun, delightful to sail and beautiful to look at.

In 1967 he produced a design for something quite revolutionary: a modern version of a vessel known as a proa. Like the traditional Polynesian boats, she had one hull and one outrigger or float and no bow or stern. Instead of tacking she merely reversed her direction of travel, always keeping her one float to leeward. She had a rudder at each end which could be raised when not in use and the two masts carried identical sails, the booms of which could be swung through 180 degrees. She was 40-foot-long and was christened *Cheers*. As Newick put it: "It sure helps if you can leave one hull at home."

In 1968 Dick Newick entered this creation for the four-yearly Observer Single Handed Transatlantic Race from Plymouth in England to Newport on Rhode Island in the USA; the race is known to everyone as the OSTAR. Initially the race organising committee, the Royal Western Yacht Club of Plymouth, refused to accept this entry as they had never seen anything like it before and doubted its seaworthiness for a transatlantic voyage. This did not put off the team behind the project who continued with sea trials, despite the vessel capsizing in the lee of Guadeloupe (just what the organising committee feared would happen). Full of confidence Tom Follett, a very experienced American skipper who had been chosen for the job, set off to sail across the Atlantic to Plymouth. On arrival he was delighted to be told the entry would be accepted after all, so impressed were the committee by this voyage.

Heavy weather dominated the race that year and, despite this, *Cheers* finished in a fast time of 27 days, beaten only by two monohull yachts both over 50-foot long. *Cheers* was third overall and the first multihull to finish. No other proa has ever finished an OSTAR and later, after a number of accidents with them, they were banned from taking part.

Cheers made history and is now owned by a French couple who have restored her to her original condition and the French Government, where long distance yacht racing has become a major sport and a near religion, has declared the boat to be an historical monument. Richard Boehmer, a nautical historian, has written 'I think it was not just the speed but also the beauty of Newick's boats that so strongly stimulated the aesthetic sensibilities of the French.'

Back in St Croix, Newick turned his hand to the design of what became his most famous creation, a 46-foot trimaran to be called *Three Cheers*. She was beautiful to look at, with gentle curves and an exaggerated sheer to the main hull and amas (the Polynesian word used by Newick for the outriggers or floats). The three hulls were held together by a steeply curved turtle deck giving great strength and allowing spacious accommodation below. She was painted primrose yellow and was a joy to sail, seemingly skimming across the water like a large yellow bird. *Three Cheers* was yawl rigged and displaced only three tons, a staggeringly light weight in those days for a 46-foot yacht and she was sufficiently well balanced not to require any form of self-steering.

Years later when asked where he got the ideas for the 140 or so designs he completed Newick, who believed in reincarnation, said that he had been a Polynesian boat builder in a previous life. He described the Polynesians' 4,000-year-old canoes as the wave of the future and said that the ancient and modern multi-hulled boats shared a theme – simplicity. He used to say that it took a good and creative person to do something simply and he famously remarked that one could only ever have in a boat two out of the three qualities: speed, comfort or cost. Newick died in California at the age of 87 on 28 August 2013.

Dick Newick and his colleague Jim Morris, who funded the 'Cheers' project, entered *Three Cheers* into the 1972 OSTAR. The tough American Tom Follett was again chosen as skipper to sail the trimaran across the Atlantic and then to sail her in the OSTAR. Follett sailed the 4,000 miles from the Virgin Islands to Plymouth in 24 days. In the weeks before the race the 'Cheers' team again made a big splash and the photogenic yellow trimaran was the centre of attraction.

One person who accepted the offer of a day sail on board *Three Cheers*, soon after her arrival, was a Royal Marine Captain called Michael McMullen, known to everyone as Mike. Mike who, up until then, had been extremely prejudiced against multihulls was smitten by this sail and said that he would never forget the experience. *Three Cheers* reached a speed of 18 knots in 15 knots of wind and he could not comprehend how a yacht could travel so fast. From that day onward his fascination with these unconventional yachts began.

*

Mike McMullen was an ebullient, larger-than-life, character: an extrovert who was instantly liked by everyone he met. He was strong, tough as nails and totally unafraid of anything. A 'last one round the Horn's a cissy' type.

Mike was born in 1943, the same year as myself. We were both born into naval families and we both spent time in Malta and later in Paris, where our fathers were stationed.

Mike's father was the renowned naval officer Colin McMullen, who died in 1991 aged 84. He was the gunnery officer on the battleship *HMS Prince of Wales* when the ship was engaged in the dramatic pursuit of the German battleship *Bismark*. Later he was probably the last man to leave the *Prince of Wales*, when she was sunk by the Japanese in one of the Royal Navy's greatest disasters of the Second World War. There were 327 fatalities which included the Admiral and the Captain. He went on to captain a destroyer on several Arctic convoys (as did my father). After the war he served in the Mediterranean and in 1954 was in charge of the salvage operation to recover the wreck of the Comet airliner that crashed off Naples. I recall Commodore McMullen, as he then was, when he was stationed in Paris in 1954 living on a Dutch barge, the *Bries*, moored on the River Seine. I well remember dining on board the barge with my father when there was a thump and scuffle on deck and the Commodore's steward came below to say he had rescued a body floating past the barge. "Well just throw the bloody thing back," the Commodore roared. Coincidentally and later in her life, my aunt Monica (mentioned in Chapter 1) had a long love affair with a subsequent owner of the *Bries* and they spent many happy years living aboard and cruising the Mediterranean until the owner died.

Mike was educated at Marlborough College and started sailing at a young age. Mike learnt his seamanship on board his father's and uncle's yachts during his school holidays. Later Mike became an active member of the Royal Cruising Club: a somewhat exclusive set up whose members pride themselves on making long voyages under sail and keeping traditional seamanship alive, combined with lots of ship-visiting and socialising when in harbour. A number of the sailors mentioned in this book were members and Mike's father was Commodore of the club from 1972 to 1977.

Mike was more an action man than an academic and, as a first job on leaving school, worked as a labourer on the construction of the road bridge high above the Firth of Forth in Scotland. Subsequently he joined the Royal Marines where he was commissioned. He later commanded a climbing wing and was a Commando Arctic Warfare instructor in North Norway.

Mike's first yacht was a diminutive 25-foot Contessa 26 called *Binkie* in which he and fellow Marine officer Martin Read took part in the second Two Handed Round Britain and Ireland Race in 1970.

This race, held every four years, had been conceived, along with the OSTAR, by the maverick inventive genius (and also ex Royal Marine officer) Blondie Hasler of 'Cockleshell Heroes' fame and much else beside. Blondie first had the idea for a single handed transatlantic race back in 1956 and, after several false starts, issued a press release in 1959 which said:

Described by one experienced yachtsman as 'the most sporting event of the century', a transatlantic race for single-handed sailing boats will start from the south coast of England on Saturday 11 June 1960 and will finish in the approaches to New York at least a month later.

Blondie then set about finding a yacht club to organise the race and a newspaper to sponsor it. The Royal Western Yacht Club in Plymouth agreed to start the race and the Sunday newspaper, the *Observer*, agreed to sponsor it. Thus was born the sport of single- or short-handed ocean racing. This has become a world-wide sport and now involves large multi-million pound heavily sponsored boats (mainly French) racing at ever increasing speeds around the oceans of the world, often with a single person on board.

After the first two OSTARs, which were held at four year-ly intervals, Blondie came up with the idea for another race: a two-handed race round the British Isles and Ireland with only four stops, each stop of exactly 48 hours. Many regard this race as a sterner test for boats and of seamanship than the OSTAR. The race, again organised by the Royal Western Yacht Club, starts from Plymouth and is divided into four legs with stops in Crosshaven in Ireland, Castle Bay in the Hebrides, Lerwick in the Shetlands and Lowestoft (the first race stopped at Harwich). No boat is allowed to leave a stop within 48 hours of its arrival. The course takes the boats outside the whole of Great Britain and Ireland and all outlying islands, including St Kilda and the Shetland Islands but excludes Rockall.

The first race was held in 1966 and was a great success. It was won by an innovative trimaran called *Toria* designed, built and sailed by Derek Kelsall. Of the sixteen starters, ten finished and the first six places were taken by multihulls.

For the second race, held in 1970, there were 25 starters of which 20 finished. Amongst the assembled fleet were such well-known names as Robin Knox-Johnston, sailing a huge 71-foot monohull and the likeable American Phil Weld in a Kelsall-designed trimaran *Trumpeter*. There was a strong Royal Naval and Royal Marine contingent, including Mike and Martin Read in *Binkie*, the smallest yacht in the fleet. They were one of the most popular crews, enjoying the hospitality at every stop and making everyone feel that there was no place in the world where they would rather be. They finished in a little over 27 days and won the race on handicap. A Contessa 26 is a tiny boat in which to circumnavigate the British Isles. They were helped on the first leg to Crosshaven by very light winds enabling *Binkie* to be rowed past several larger boats (this was allowed within the rules).

Writing after the race Mike said: 'The leg from Crosshaven to Barra was for *Binkie* certainly alarming. Once round the south west corner of Eire a westerly gale blew up which lasted the whole way to the Hebrides. In winds gusting to Force 8 we ran up the Atlantic coast of Ireland before frighteningly large seas at a very high speed. Once we were knocked flat by a sea which gave us both unfavourable impressions of the whole proceedings and in a moment of weakness I almost (not quite) wished I was with 45 Commando over in Belfast 130 miles away.'

Off Muckle Flugga, the most northerly piece of land in the British Isles, Mike and Martin sailed *Binkie* close in to the rocky headland and inside a notorious tidal race. The principal light-house keeper, Mr Tulloch, was so impressed by this tactic that he rushed to hoist and dip his ensign in tribute, saying later that he thought it was a grand piece of sailing and he had to admire the crew for their daring.

On the last lap from Lowestoft to Plymouth, whilst the leaders faced yet another gale, *Binkie* had to contend with light winds and Mike and Martin rowed from the time they were off Salcombe until they reached Plymouth. They were rewarded by winning the Daily Express Trophy for the first yacht on corrected time. First boat home in the race was the huge and heavy *Ocean Spirit* sailed by Robin Knox-Johnston and naval officer Leslie Williams. It was quite an achievement for two people to sail a boat of that size around that course through some atrocious weather.

After the Round Britain Race Mike swapped *Binkie* for a larg-er yacht, a 32-foot Contessa 32, which Mike named *Binkie II*. This particular class of yacht, of which many were built, has acquired almost legendary status for its sea-keeping qualities and they have been chosen by many long distance sailors for long voyages, often to polar and high latitude regions. Mike had *Binkie II* built aiming to win the under 35ft prize in the 1972 OSTAR.

She was launched in December 1971 and he took the sail number 45, being the number of his commando group.

The usual motley fleet began to assemble in Plymouth for the OSTAR in June 1972, ranging from the huge 128-foot staysail schooner *Vendredi Treize*, Eric Tabarly's trimaran *Pen Duick IV* in the hands of Alain Colas, down to the diminutive 19-foot *Willing Griffin*. The popular Phil Weld appeared again with his trimaran *Trumpeter*, along with Sir Francis Chichester in his latest Gipsy Moth, *Gipsy Moth V*, despite having been advised by his doctors not to take part. There were 55 starters and Mike arrived in *Binkie II* with a fierce determination to win his class.

It is always instructive before these races to walk around the assembled fleet in Millbay Dock and watch the goings on aboard and around the boats. Some would be full of fevered activity with worried looking skippers and supporters trying to get everything ready and to get bits of equipment to work. Others would be calm and ordered, with the skippers pottering around happily chatting to friends and neighbours. From this you could glean a lot as to the boat's likely success or otherwise.

The favourite, the trimaran *Pen Duick IV*, sat starkly in one corner of the dock, its aluminium structure a bit battered and bruised after Colas' recent voyage from Tahiti to Europe, mostly single-handed. She was well prepared and ready to go, with Colas refusing to talk to well-wishers, saying he was keyed up for the race and not wanting any distractions. The *Three Cheers* team could hardly have been more different. Tom Follett was his usual affable self, handing out advice to first timers and speaking to anyone who approached. Dick Newick was, as ever, polite and only too pleased to show anyone over his new creation.

Over on another side of the Dock there were several boats

holding never ending parties, one being *Binkie II* where Mike entertained his family, Royal Marine compatriots and friends from dawn to dusk.

A pre-race photograph of the OSTAR skippers shows Mike at the extreme top left corner looking confident and larger than life, shouting something at the camera with raised arms. Tom Follett, the skipper of *Three Cheers*, is sitting on the extreme bottom right of the same photograph looking away from the camera subdued, calm and pensive.

Up until this time Mike, like most yachtsmen, had not a good word to say about multihulls and Mike remembers pontificating at several yacht club bars to fellow sailors: "You will never get me out in one of those machines... unsafe... unstable... held together by bits of string... unfit to cross the Thames and bloody ugly!" Like thousands of others he was prepared to condemn, without trial, a type of vessel about which he knew nothing and had never sailed. However, as he joined the assembled craft at Plymouth before the race he became aware of the large multihull entry, mostly trimarans and he admitted to a latent curiosity about them. It was then that Mike enjoyed his day sail on board *Three Cheers*, which totally changed his attitude.

A brisk south westerly wind was blowing as the fleet sped away from the start line on Saturday 17 June 1972. Jean-Yves Terlain eased his massive 128-foot *Vendredi Treize* through the unruly spectator fleet with Gallic coolness. Phil Weld in this his first OSTAR (he was later to become a winner) sped past the big French boat in his trimaran *Trumpeter*, pursued by Mike in *Binkie II*. The competitors, after some initial strong winds in the Western Approaches, faced a lot of benign weather and on arrival at Newport most complained more of calms and fog than of gales and bad weather.

This was to be the year of the French. They captured the first three places, the winner being Alain Colas in the trimaran *Pen Duick IV*. He completed the course in 20 days. The huge three-masted schooner *Vendredi Treize* limped in the next day having had to put into Newfoundland for repairs. Disappointingly *Three Cheers* came in fifth taking 27 days.

Before the start Tom Follett had stated that he could reach Newport in 16 days but after 25 days the race organisers began to wonder what had happened; in those days there was virtually no contact with the shore, few had transmitting radios and no one had monitoring beacons. A look of concern began to appear on the faces of the waiting team. In the week before Follett arrived a heavy fog descended on the area and most thought or hoped that he was just becalmed. Eventually on day 27 *Three Cheers* arrived unannounced; the yellow bird looming suddenly out of the fog having been missed by the Coastguard and by the awaiting boat on the finish line.

Follett reported having had very bad winds and on one day he made only 31 miles; he had lots of poor daily runs of 60, 70 or 80 miles. This was from a boat easily capable of making 300 miles a day in the right conditions. Follett, who took the minimum of stores with him, nearly ran out of water and supplies. At the end he had a gallon of water left, two cans of soup, one can of carrots and a few crisps. He also reported that he was nearly run down by a cargo ship on the second day out from Plymouth.

Mike nearly achieved his objective of winning the under 35-foot prize, completing the course in just over 31 days. He was less than four days behind the much faster and larger *Three Cheers*. Mike and *Binkie II* were beaten in their class only by a brilliant

64

performance from the Frenchman Alain Gliksman in his 35-foot-long *Toucan* who came in eighth overall in 28 days, having had an extremely wet and uncomfortable crossing. *Toucan* was basically an open day boat designed for sailing on the Swiss lakes. She was little more than an overgrown dinghy onto which Alain had built a deck and a small cabin. It was all he could afford.

As was to be expected, on arrival Mike was greeting everyone, sipping champagne with abandon, before the fenders were over the side. Within minutes he had a party going and this was at nine o'clock in the morning. 32 days alone at sea had not dimmed his *joie de vivre*.

Binkie II took thirteenth place overall. Mike took the northern route after leaving Land's End but was frustrated by calms and fog. The only real problem he had was with a deck fitting holding the foot of the forestay, which broke in a force 7 wind. It took him several hours to repair. Before crossing the finishing line, he sailed very close in to Martha's Vineyard, a risky venture even with good visibility. He saw nothing in the fog, save for one channel buoy, navigating on echo-soundings and rough bearings from his direction finding radio. The local Coastguard Chief, and an expert on those dangerous waters, said glumly that Mike shouldn't boast too much about what he had done. Despite all his bonhomie, Mike was serious about the risks involved in this sort of racing and admitted to fear when amongst icebergs. He recounted how frightened he was when nearly run down in thick fog near the Brenton Tower.

The saddest story of the 1972 race was that of Sir Frances Chichester and his *Gipsy Moth V*. Sir Francis gave up within a week due to ill health and started to head back toward Plymouth. Confusion then arose and a message he passed back to an RAF

Nimrod aircraft was misinterpreted. A full rescue operation was mounted and a French weather ship, *France II*, hoping to help out the old mariner, came too close and broke the yacht's mizzen mast making it almost impossible for the yacht to be sailed home. *HMS Salisbury*, a Royal Navy frigate, was despatched with Sir Francis's son Giles on board, together with a friend and a rigging expert. They were put aboard the stricken yacht which they sailed home. Sadly, *France II*, having disabled *Gipsy Moth V*, then collided with an American yacht called *Lefteria*, the crew of which were also trying to find and help the single-hander. The yacht sank, four of her crew were rescued and one body recovered. The other six crew members went missing. In all seven lives

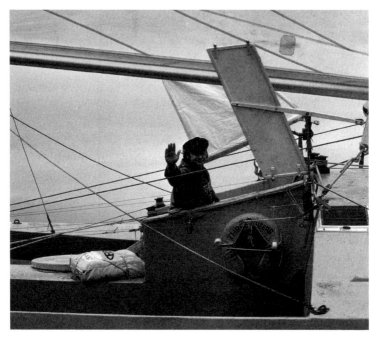

Mike McMullen on board Three Cheers

were lost. A sad end to a chapter of misplaced well-intentions. This turned out to be Sir Francis's last voyage and he died in his bed before the year was out.

After the race, Mike approached Dick Newick to enquire if *Three Cheers* might be for sale. The answer was positive and Mike set about finding the funds to buy her. A throwaway line in Mike's book *Multihull Seamanship* gave the clue as to how the purchase of *Three Cheers* was arranged. In the forward to his book Mike gave thanks 'to the kindness of his father's cousin, Paul Mellon, for buying and lending him *Three Cheers*.'

The family relationship between the McMullens and the immensely rich Mellon family goes back two generations. In 1900 Andrew Mellon, founder of the dynasty, married a nineteen-year-old English girl, Nora McMullen, who was Mike's father's aunt. The marriage was a disaster but they had two children. One, their son Paul, was born in 1907 and he inherited his father's wealth. By 1972 he was one of the richest men in America. Mike, or his father, approached him and he agreed to buy *Three Cheers* and allow Mike to sail and look after her as if she was his own.

Mike sailed the boat back across the Atlantic to England and based her in Lymington in Hampshire, where he lived with his recently married wife, Lizzie. During the next few years he sailed *Three Cheers* long and hard around the United Kingdom, with further passages abroad. The sight of this yellow bird skimming the waters of the Solent became well known. He began to learn how to handle multihulls, which behave very differently from single-hulled yachts, and how to get the best out of *Three Cheers*. Mike entered her in the 1973 Crystal Trophy, the premier UK race for multihulls, with a course from the Solent to Cherbourg, then down channel to the Wolf Rock off the southern tip of Cornwall and back to Cowes. *Three Cheers* won.

He took the trimaran on a family cruise to Spain, despite her minimal accommodation. In Mike's book *Multihull Seamanship* there are several photographs of *Three Cheers* on this cruise, one showing her hauled up on a Spanish beach and another motoring into a rocky bay.

In 1974 Mike and *Three Cheers* were joined in England by another Newick-designed trimaran, the 60-foot *Gulf Streamer*. She was built at great cost in America for Massachusetts newspaper proprietor Phil Weld and sailed over to England by him earlier that year. She was basically a blown up *Three Cheers* but with three crossbeams taking the place of the turtle deck. She was blisteringly fast, extremely comfortable, extremely well equipped and sailed hard by Weld. In later years he became a popular figure and a good friend to many people in England, including myself.

It was the intention of both skippers to enter their trimarans in the forthcoming Round Britain and Ireland Race which was due to start in June of that year. The two boats sparred with each other during the early part of the 1974 season and there is an iconic and much reproduced Beken photograph of the two Newick trimarans close reaching at speed in the Solent. Both boats took part in several short races and *Gulf Streamer* won the 1974 Crystal Trophy with ease.

The 1974 Round Britain Race was a glittering affair with 61 starters from six nations. Robin Knox-Johnston returned, this time at the helm of a fast 70-foot catamaran, *British Oxygen*. Phil Weld and Mike (crewed again by his fellow marine Martin Read) were there with their Newick boats, as was Alain Colas with the old trimaran *Pen Duick IV*, now named *Manureva*. She was looking tired, battered and bruised having recently returned from a solo round the world trip. There were some new Kelsall-designed trimarans, notably David Palmer (then the news editor of the *Financial Times*) with his salmon pink *FT* and Nick Keig, a jovial photographer from the Isle of Mann, with *Three Legs of Mann*, a self-built boat which proved extremely fast.

Light winds predominated during the first leg to Crosshaven and *British Oxygen* arrived first, followed closely by *Three Cheers*. *Manureva* could only come in tenth, a position from which Colas never recovered; from then on merely following the leaders around the course. He said afterwards that he had underestimated the quality of the opposition and that he should have removed much of the heavy equipment used in his circumnavigation. *Gulf Streamer* came in fourth, with another trimaran, *Triple Arrow*, coming in third. On the second leg to Barra, Mike and *Three Cheers* came in one hour behind *Gulf Streamer*, who was now second overall to *British Oxygen*. The slower boats experienced much bad weather on this leg. On the third leg to Lerwick in the Shetland Islands the leaders had favourable weather and *Three Cheers* came in first.

Disaster nearly struck *Three Cheers* on the next leg south to Lowestoft. She was powering to windward over a dull grey lumpy North Sea when Mike went forward to change a headsail in a strengthening wind. He was pitched overboard from a heaving deck. Being on the foredeck of a multihull working to windward at speed is akin to being bounced up and down on a trampoline. *Gulf Streamer* was in sight two miles off and *British Oxygen* was to seaward of them. It was the crew's normal practice on *Three Cheers*, when changing a headsail going to windward (virtually no-one had furling headsails in those days), to slow the boat as much as possible by pinching her close to the wind so that movement is at a minimum. This is what they did and Mike went forward and changed the sails without a hitch. Mike hoisted the new smaller sail, whilst Martin at the helm paid the boat off and started to winch in the sheet. However, the sheets had fouled themselves into a 'steel ball' so Mike dropped the sail and, without thinking, rushed forward to clear the jam. By now the boat had accelerated and was charging to windward at about nine knots. Within seconds Mike was pitched overboard. Luckily, Mike still had hold of a line and only half of him was in the water. Martin, seeing what had happened, shoved the helm hard over which brought the boat into the wind and stopped her. Martin rushed forward to help Mike back aboard. But, by the time he had reached him, the pull of the water had got at Mike, he could no longer hold on and he was gone – Martin could only see a flash of yellow in the grey sea.

The next thing Mike remembers was a painful bang on his left thigh as he went underneath the boat and hit the rudder at about 5 knots. He came up on the other side to find the boat hove to on the other tack with staysail aback some 30 metres upwind. Luckily she was drifting downwind faster than Mike was, both drifting in the same direction. As Mike put it in his book, 'like a true lady, she drifted straight back to me.'

The problem now was that although Mike was holding onto the lee float, he could not haul himself aboard and the leeway the boat was making was pushing Mike under. Mike, who was a very large man, was wearing seaboots, longjohns, trousers, shirt, two sweaters, oilskin trousers with braces and a fisherman's smock that came down to his knees. They concluded the only way to get Mike on board was for Martin to winch him up on a halyard.

Martin lowered all sails, other than the mizzen, to try to slow her down. Martin then got a rope around Mike and winched him aboard. It took them a long time to get going again. By this time *British Oxygen* was away and over the horizon.

Mike admitted later that he had nearly drowned and, had Martin not been so quick thinking to crash stop the boat but had adopted the more traditional procedure of sailing the boat off in a circle to bring her back alongside the casualty, Mike thinks he would have been long gone. He said, "I was swallowing water so fast in the rough sea and, weighed down by clothing, I could not get out of, I felt that drowning could not have been too many minutes away."

One must question why Mike and Martin, both experienced sailors, were not wearing safety harnesses or life jackets. If Mike had worn a harness, he would not have been separated from the boat and Martin could have winched Mike aboard from the fore-deck. A life jacket would have given Mike sufficient buoyancy to stay afloat until winched back on board. It is easy to criticise and it must be remembered that life jackets were little used in the 1970s and safety harnesses were often only donned at night or in really bad weather. We are all a little wiser nowadays and Mike admitted that he had learnt the hard way and was lucky to survive.

This accident allowed *British Oxygen* to get clear away and she arrived in Lowestoft first, some nine hours ahead. The final leg back to Plymouth was sailed in light conditions which slowed *British Oxygen* somewhat. Robin Knox-Johnston sailed her over the finishing line in first place in an elapsed time of just over 18 days. *Three Cheers* came in second only one and a half hours later. One speculates as to who would have been the winner had *Three*

Cheers not lost time sorting out their problems after the man over-board incident. Whatever the position, it was a great piece of sailing by Mike and Martin in a boat much smaller than *British Oxygen. Gulf Streamer*, also a much larger and faster boat, came in third over two hours later.

Between 1974 and 1976, Mike continued to sail *Three Cheers* both in local races and on family cruises. In 1975, as part of his work up for the OSTAR, he took *Three Cheers*, with his wife Lizzie and a friend as crew, on a six-week cruise around the Western Isles of Scotland. They left the River Severn in May, where Mike had had much work done to 'civilize' *Three Cheers* – he widened the bunks, installed such luxuries as seats and a table and fitted a proper marine toilet (Lizzie had decided it was between her or the black bucket if she was to live on board for six weeks!). They reached St Kilda in good weather, anchoring in Village Bay, then they attempted a landing on the uninhabited Flannan Islands, scene of an unsolved tragedy in 1900 when the entire crew of three lighthouse keepers disappeared without trace. Bad weather prevented landing but they went on to visit North Rona, another uninhabited island deep into the north Atlantic. This cruise would have been an achievement for a well-equipped cruising yacht with a full crew but for a light weight racing trimaran it was outstanding.

In this period Mike also completed work on his only published book entitled *Multihull Seamanship* which was published in 1976 with a foreword by Sir Robin Knox-Johnston. Whilst somewhat over reliant on the design and attributes of, and his experiences with, *Three Cheers*, the only multihull Mike had ever sailed in earnest, the book contains much of interest and much good advice. The sections on 'Accidents and Safety' and 'Heavy Weather' are of particular interest in the light of what may or may not have happened to Mike on his last trip in *Three Cheers* later that year.

There now occurred one of those strange coincidences that kept cropping up during my research for this book. I discovered in a discussion on an internet forum a reference to the fact that at some stage prior to the 1976 OSTAR Mike McMullen took the old irascible sea-dog H W 'Bill' Tilman (see the next Chapter) for a spin in *Three Cheers*. One can hardly think of a less likely meeting. The old mountaineer and ocean adventurer used to sailing lumbering heavy and out of date pilot cutters and the young brash ex-Marine commando showing off his almost weightless primrose yellow super-fast sailing machine. The web blog states that Mike invited Tilman and his crew out for a sail after an evening spent in a pub and on board Tilman's last boat, the decrepit and decaying pilot cutter *Baroque*.

It turned out that Tilman liked Mike a lot and actually strongly approved of *Three Cheers*, saying that she was just what a boat should be: small, simple rig, sensible accommodation, easy to manage, fast and seaworthy. But of course, he continued, no good for what he liked to do as she was unable to carry a crew of five or to work through pack ice. He said that, if he did what Mike was doing, then *Three Cheers* was the boat he would have had.

So we come to the 1976 OSTAR and the tragedy that led to Mike's final voyage. That year's race was immersed in controversy from the outset. Following on from the 1972 race (and the 128-foot-long *Vendredi Treize*) there was much discussion by the organisers as to whether or how to control the size of entrants. Blondie Hasler wanted an upper size limit of 65 feet. Others wanted to impose a time penalty on boats of over 50 feet. In the event the organisers, probably mistakenly, did no such thing but, instead, divided the fleet into three classes – the Jester Class for boats less than 28 feet on the waterline, the Gipsy Moth Class for boats less than 46 feet on the waterline and the Pen Duick Class for yachts bigger than this. There was no upper size limit.

Alain Colas entered the massive 236-foot *Club Mediterranee* amid much controversy (as described in more detail in Chapter 5). When *Club Mediterranee* arrived in Plymouth she astounded all who saw her, especially when comparing her with the smallest entry, *Spirit of Surprise*, a 25-foot modified racing Hellcat catamaran, designed for afternoon racing on inland or inshore waters. The on-board accommodation was two slots in the hulls into which the skipper could slide into a reclining, but not lying, position! (The skipper Ambrogio Fogar, a controversial figure at the best of times, actually made it as far as the Azores before retiring.)

The pre-race jamboree in Plymouth was characterised by the usual chaos on some entries, calm on others and much partying on others. Notable amongst the latter group was, of course, Mike on *Three Cheers*, and a new entrant to these races, the gregarious yacht designer Angus Primrose on his own designed boat, a Moody 33, *Demon Demo*.

The race that year was extremely competitive and all the big names in short-handed racing turned up. Eric Tabarly was there with his *Pen Duick VI*, a huge and heavy 73-foot-long ketch, normally sailed by a crew of 12 or 14, and last used in a fully crewed round-the-world race. Tabarly arrived with an army (or rather French navy) of helpers and sat quietly in a corner of his cockpit saying little but occasionally issuing an order and watching it being carried out, the complete professional, unruffled, unhurried and totally self-contained.

125 yachts had been passed by the scrutineers and were readying themselves to start the race when tragedy struck. On Thursday 3 June, only 48 hours before the start, Mike had *Three Cheers* lifted out of the water onto the hard standing at Mashford's Boatyard, just across the River Tamar from where the OSTAR fleet was assembled. He wanted to set off with three clean and polished bottoms. Lizzie, his wife, was helping him and was using an electric polisher plugged into the mains electricity. She dropped the polisher into a puddle of shallow water underneath the boat and without thinking stooped down to pick it up. She was electrocuted and collapsed.

Lizzie was taken to nearby Stonehouse Hospital. Richard Clifford, also a Marine and Mike's friend and fellow OSTAR competitor, was one of the first to hear the news and sped on his bicycle to the hospital where he joined Martin Read (Mike's co-skipper in earlier races) and some other friends in the emergency ward where they were trying to resuscitate Lizzie. This was unsuccessful and she was pronounced dead.

It is hard to get across the huge impact this tragedy had on the close knit group of sailors assembled in Plymouth, a group highly emotionally charged anyway with the start just hours away. Richard Clifford volunteered to break the news to all the others and cycled back to Millbay Dock. That evening's entertainment was subdued and everyone was hushed and shocked.

People were devastated. Within hours it was proposed that a trophy should be created in Lizzie's memory and donations were forthcoming from all sides. Thus the Lizzie McMullen Memorial Trophy was born, a silver plated model of *Three Cheers*. It has been awarded ever since to the first multihull to finish an

OSTAR.

Lizzie's funeral took place the following day. With great courage Mike decided that Lizzie would have wanted him to continue with the race, which he had a real chance of winning despite the intense competition. Everyone was sure Lizzie would have wanted him to go.

The next day Mike set off with the rest of the fleet.

The start took place in light weather, just as well with the huge *Club Mediterranee* threading its way amongst an armada of press and spectator boats. One competitor, Henk Jukkema, took an iconic photograph of Mike sitting calmly at the helm of *Three Cheers* as he made his way to the start.

Late the next day *Three Cheers* was sighted off Galley Head on the south west coast of Ireland. A local fisherman spoke to Mike as he sailed past in light weather. This was the last ever sighting of the trimaran.

Twenty-four days after the start, multihulls smaller and slower than *Three Cheers* began to cross the finishing line in Newport, led by Mike Birch in the diminutive *Third Turtle*. Fears began to grow for McMullen's safety. It should be emphasised that, in those days, competitors did not have any form of tracking device and few boats were fitted with long distance radio transmitters. Once a competitor had sailed over the horizon he had to all intents and purposes disappeared until spotted by another ship or until land was reached.

After thirty-three days at sea, Richard Clifford crossed the finishing line in 30th place, to find Gill McMullen, Mike's mother, still anxiously waiting for him. Lizzie's mother had also made the trip to Newport. A Royal Navy ship had been diverted to search for the trimaran. Everyone in Newport remained very positive.

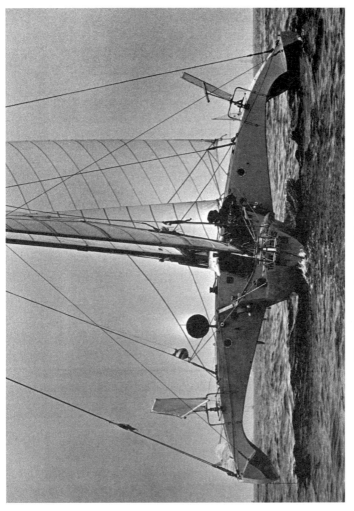

Three Cheers at the start of the 1976 OSTAR

"Oh, Mike will turn up," they said. Projected courses for *Three Cheers* were drawn up and computerised models for the drift of a stricken yacht in the North Atlantic were made. An aerial search based on these was carried out but this produced no sightings.

Most people think that Mike's disappearance stemmed from his determination to win the event for his late wife, so he threw caution to the winds and 'just went for it'. No one will ever know what really happened. There was gale after gale during the race. Maybe Mike flipped *Three Cheers*, maybe he was in a collision with another boat or with an iceberg or maybe the boat just broke up, driven too hard.

Before the race there were the inevitable discussions between competitors as to what course to take for Newport. Basically there are three available routes. The southerly route is the longest but gives one the best weather. The rhumb line route, favoured by most competitors, is shorter and should keep one south of the worst weather. The great circle route is the shortest but takes one far north into the region of storms, ice and fog and close to Newfoundland. In theory one is then north of the depressions rushing east across the Atlantic getting favourable winds for much of the time but with a greater danger from ice and fog.

I believe that Mike took a route far to the north and that somewhere up there, whilst sailing hard, he was simply overwhelmed by bad weather which flipped the multihull, which subsequently broke up.

The only evidence for this is the finding of two pieces of wreckage from *Three Cheers* near Iceland. The first piece was some wreckage found in July 1977, washed ashore four and a half miles west of Iceland's Thoras River. This consisted of part of a trimaran's ama or float together with part of a sail with the sail number 9 (*Three Cheers* sail number for the race was 99). The wreckage was positively identified as part of *Three Cheers*. This finding was not reported to the UK until three years later, in October 1980 (relations between Iceland and the UK were not good at that time with the cod wars in full spate).

Another part of *Three Cheers* was found in 1980. In a somewhat ironic twist this was reported to the UK just days before the start of the 1980 OSTAR. An Icelandic trawler off the south coast of Iceland had dredged up a piece of wreckage which had some electronic instruments attached. The serial numbers of these were identified by the manufacturers, Brookes & Gatehouse, as being those installed on *Three Cheers*.

No other trace of the boat or of Mike McMullen has ever been found.

Chapter 4

The Last Voyage of Simon Richardson and Bill Tilman and the Loss of *En Avant* in the South Atlantic (1977)

The loss of an old converted Dutch steel tug in the South Atlantic in 1997 and the loss of six young men would have made few headlines in the UK press had it not been for the fact that also on board was the famous 80-year-old indomitable mountaineer, adventurer, explorer and ocean voyager, Major H W 'Bill' Tilman.

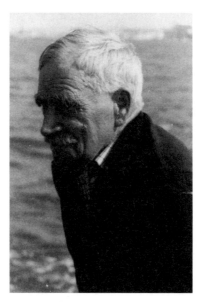

Bill Tilman on board En Avant

Little of this story and the reason why Tilman, at the age of 80, had shipped as crew on a vessel headed for Antarctica, owned and skippered by a young Englishman, Simon Richardson, would ever have been known had not Simon's mother, Dorothy, written an account of the incident and of her son's brief life entitled *The Quest of Simon Richardson*.

I first met Bill Tilman in 1961 when he answered an advertisement I had placed in *Yachting Monthly* seeking a sailing adventure during my gap year before University. He asked me if I wanted to join his Bristol Channel Pilot Cutter *Mischief* as part of the crew for a proposed trip to Baffin Island. I was intrigued and spent some time on board *Mischief* with the old man in Lymington and helped him with the fitting out of the boat for his trip. To my eternal regret I eventually turned down his offer. At that time Tilman was little known and to my youthful and ignorant eye I was somewhat appalled at the condition of *Mischief* and the state of some of her sailing gear. I could see straight through the topside seams in places and there were many rotten areas in her planks and frames.

Another reason for my turning down his offer was that Tilman did not envisage returning to the UK until November and I was due to start at St Andrews University in Scotland that September. Had I had more guts I should have accepted Tilman's rather vague offer to put me ashore somewhere in Greenland in good time to get me back for the start of the university term. When I did get to St Andrews I was told that I could have met up, and had a lift back home, with a student expedition from the university which was spending the summer in the research hut which St Andrews maintained on the west coast of Greenland. Tilman and *Mischief* later that year did in fact meet up with them. Dr

81

Harold Drever, who was leading the expedition, was an old friend of Tilman's and he later taught me geology at St Andrews.

A year later, Dr Drever told me that he was surprised that I was not on board *Mischief* when they met up in Greenland as Tilman had told him he was going to have a St Andrews student on board for the trip to Baffin Island. To this day I don't know why Tilman never said any of this to me but he was never a good communicator and maybe he thought that it wasn't his place to assist me in my decision whether to go or not. But it was a crying shame.

Tilman and his exploits will be well known to many readers of this book. What will not be so well known is that on a voyage to Greenland in 1973 on the decrepit pilot cutter *Baroque* (described in Tilman's book *Ice With Everything*) Tilman shipped with him, as part of the usual motley crew, a young Englishman called Simon Richardson.

Simon was 20 years old, the son of a Southampton solicitor. He was educated privately at Winchester College and had spent a year reading civil engineering but left his college after a year. He was impatient, wanted to start living his own life and was not really academically minded. He was extremely practical and mechanically inventive and preferred a life of action using his hands.

To gain sailing experience he signed on for several long-distance yacht delivery trips and then fell in with a man doing up an old German E boat in Italy. Simon helped him for a while, then took passage on a boat travelling through the French canals. Back in England he applied to join the British Antarctic Survey. Before he received a reply, he saw an advertisement in *The Times*, inserted by Tilman, seeking crew for a voyage to Greenland.

Simon jumped at the chance.

Simon joined *Baroque* at Mylor on the River Fal in Cornwall in May 1973 and soon established himself as the most capable member of the crew. His mechanical and inventive skills were soon put to use as the boat was, basically, falling apart. It was mainly through Simon's efforts that *Baroque* made it to Greenland at all.

Tilman was renowned as an irascible and difficult character regularly falling out with his crews, who generally ended up loathing him and vowing never to ship with him again. (On one earlier voyage in his first ship, *Mischief*, the crew mutinied in South America and walked ashore.) With Simon, however it was different. Tilman saw something in the young man, appreciated his efforts and attitude, and a relationship of sorts developed between them. Tilman may well have seen something of himself in Simon's attitude if not directly in his character. Tilman said later that he had picked a winner in Simon and he found him active, energetic, knowledgeable about boats and engines and a thorough seaman. Simon also got on with the other crew members and the voyage became one of Tilman's happiest and most successful, despite the condition of *Baroque*. She leaked like a sieve, the port chain plates soon pulled out, the sails were old and rotten, the engine kept failing and the bulwarks up forward disintegrated. The crew pumped incessantly.

Simon kept and wrote a journal of the voyage which he intended one day to publish in book form. Dorothy, his mother, published the journal in full in her book about Simon. It is one of the few (and best) accounts written, other than by Tilman himself, of what voyaging with the old man was really like. It makes fascinating reading.

It is not easy to get to the bottom of Simon's character at this stage of his life. One of Tilman's biographer's, Tim Madge, refers to Simon's slipshod arrogance. Simon had a great belief in himself and his ability to achieve impossible aims. He was also very much in thrall to the old man, believing himself some kind of heir to Tilman's ambitions. It was this which made Simon so obsessive about having Tilman with him on his own forthcoming voyage, which proved fatal for both of them. Simon's mother, Dorothy, compares Simon directly with Tilman and said that she could understand anyone who found her son tiresome, slapdash, undisciplined and loutish.

On Simon's return to the UK in October 1973, he was, for a while, at a loss as to what to do next but he had definitely caught the 'polar' bug and began to plan how to bring this about. After some casual work Simon received an invitation from Tilman to join him on a trip to Spitzbergen planned for 1974. Simon accepted but a few weeks later his father died following a stroke and Simon, deeply affected, felt he should get a proper job. He withdrew from the proposed trip. Simon soon obtained a job in Scotland building a new harbour and plant for offshore oil rigs. This was dangerous but well paid work during which he learnt his skills as a welder. In April 1975 he was appointed Assistant Marine Controller, even though he was one of the youngest employees.

In October 1974, just as work on the harbour was coming to an end, Simon suffered a serious injury to one of his legs. He was knocked off the quay by a crane and landed on the steel deck of a ship 17 feet below. His right leg was shattered just above the ankle. He was in hospital in Greenock for a month, where he was told that he would never walk again unaided. Convalescing back at home in Hampshire he had further treatment and after a few weeks was, in fact, able to start walking with the help of crutches.

Simon was now 23 and, during his recuperation, began to develop the plan he had first dreamt up on his Greenland trip: to sail to Smith Island in Antarctica, part of the South Shetland Islands, and to climb Mount Foster, the highest mountain in the region. Such an expedition was fully in the tradition of Tilman's voyages and had, in fact, been attempted by Tilman himself in 1966, in *Mischief.* That was the only voyage on which Tilman had lost a man overboard.

The main problem, however, was that Simon did not have a boat and had little money. Simon thought long and hard about this and reckoned that, by using his welding skills, he could afford to buy and convert one of the decommissioned working vessels which were being offered for sale in Holland. He bought for £750, sight unseen, an 18 metre steel tug which had been involved in a serious marine accident, leaving the boat sunk and one crew member dead. She had been refloated but much work was needed. She had no engine, no accommodation and would need to be adapted to take a mast and sails. The boat was called *En Avant.*

She was 64 feet long, 15 feet wide and drew 5 feet. She had been built in Rotterdam in 1942 by Dutch slave labour. Simon designed a gaff rig for her and planned accommodation for a crew of eight.

Simon moved to Holland and started work on the boat, even though his leg was still in plaster and he needed two sticks to walk. He lived aboard a friend's boat. He installed a second hand diesel engine which he had brought over from England, fitted out some basic accommodation below, added a mast for a gaff rigged sail and welded on a hollow steel box keel to help with her sailing ability.

A Dutch optician, who Simon had befriended after visiting his surgery to have a small piece of steel removed from his eye, accompanied Simon when bringing *En Avant* from Holland back to Southampton. They had a hair-raising trip, which showed up some of the boat's weaknesses.

Back in England, work continued throughout the winter. Simon had, by this stage, asked Bill Tilman if he wished to join the expedition. Tilman, after a disastrous voyage in *Baroque* to Spitzbergen during which he had been forced to abandon his boat in Iceland, went to visit Simon and the tug. He remained non-committal but Simon was adamant that he wanted Tilman on board.

By April work was as complete as it ever would be but Simon still had no crew, except for an old school friend who had agreed to come along. He was Mark Johnson, a merchant seaman. Tilman was away bringing *Baroque* back from Iceland and had still not made a decision. *En Avant* had to leave by late July if they were to get to Smith Island before the onset of the Antarctic winter. Simon put an advertisement in The Times – 'crew wanted for Antarctic voyage' – which elicited 168 replies over a four-day period. From these Simon selected three, Rod Coatman, Robert Toombs and Charles Williams. Simon refused to consider any of the many women who replied in anticipation of Tilman, who would certainly not have approved of females on board, joining him. Later, an American climber Joe Dittamore agreed to come; he said he knew of a New Zealand climber who could join them in the Falkland Islands.

In May, Tilman arrived back in England, sold *Baroque* and

told Simon he would like to join them. It was to be Tilman's 80th birthday that year and Simon remembered a night watch discussion during his voyage in *Baroque* when Tilman expressed his wish to spend his upcoming birthday at sea in polar waters. Tilman probably knew that the recent trip back from Iceland was the last voyage he would make in his own boat.

The question arises as to why Tilman, a superb seaman, would agree to go to sea in such a seemingly unseaworthy vessel. The answer probably lies in the fact that, by then, Tilman had little to look forward to. He could no longer command his own vessel, his beloved sister with whom he had shared his house in Barmouth had recently died, as had his favourite dog. He was finding it difficult to walk the fells and hills above his house. How else could he now get to sea and what better way to celebrate his life than by spending his birthday on an expedition to Antarctica? If he ever thought about the state of the ship, maybe he was willing to accept the risk as reward for one last adventure.

Even after the conversion, the *En Avant* remained extremely tender. She had very low freeboard and no guardrails fitted around the sides. She rolled excessively. She had very poor sailing qualities, which were never properly tested before the departure. Simon had originally planned for the hollow welded-on box keel to be filled with pig iron but this was never done. Apart from the engine, and whatever water and fuel the boat carried, she had no other ballast.

En Avant departed Southampton on 9 August 1977, with seven people on board. Tilman soon learnt to fit in and became quite fond of the young crew and their ways, and never interfered with the running of the ship. *En Avant* reached the Canary Islands at the end of August after a relatively easy downwind passage.

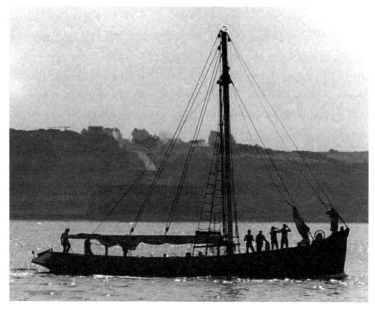

En Avant sets sail

From there they motor sailed to Rio de Janeiro on a passage which, again, never really tested the ship's sailing ability. They arrived on 29 October. Tilman reported on the passage by stating that he doubted whether he was really worth having on board. He found the gear too heavy and found it difficult to get about the wide deck with nothing to hang on to. Still, he said, it would have been a mistake to have refused Simon's invitation.

En Avant set sail in November for the Falkland Islands, where they were to pick up two New Zealand climbers. In Simon's last letter to his mother he says: 'six weeks to Port Stanley where the natives should be friendly.' He also commented that it would be interesting to see how *En Avant* liked rough weather.

En Avant never arrived in Port Stanley and was never seen

again.

A search was begun on 9 January 1978. All British Antarctic Survey ships were asked to keep a lookout and the Argentinian and Chilean air services were informed. Neither the vessel nor any of her crew nor any wreckage has ever been found.

Much speculation has been aired as to the cause of the loss. It is most likely that the boat was simply overwhelmed and foundered through stress of weather. Tugs, even when converted, are notoriously unhandy, have very low freeboard and are tender. There is also a question regarding the box keel which was merely welded to the boat's bottom and might this have fractured and torn away from the hull? Had the keel been properly through bolted, *En Avant* might have survived.

As for Tilman, there is no doubt that a bond of a sort had formed between the old sea dog and the young pretender and, before leaving, Simon had already expressed the view that Tilman might not survive the whole trip. Tilman's biographer, Tim Madge, asked whether Simon knew of the old legend that the heroes of earlier times would take young heroes with them on their avowed last voyage as a sacrifice to the Gods to ensure a welcome in Valhalla? Is this too fanciful an idea?

Tragic though the loss of *En Avant* was, it at least granted Tilman his wish not to die in his bed.

*

Since writing the above, I have learnt that two former shipmates of Tilman, Bob Comlay and John Shipton, both declined Simon's invitation to join him on *En Avant* for the voyage, as neither could afford the £500 up-front cash contribution which

Simon demanded. Bob had been on two voyages with Tilman to Greenland in the 1970s and John, who went on one trip with Tilman, is the son of the renowned explorer, Eric Shipton, with whom Tilman formed a famed partnership in the 1930s, climbing and exploring whole areas of the Himalayas previously unseen by Western eyes.

The two had a lucky escape.

Chapter 5

The Life and Loss of Alain Colas and his Trimaran *Manureva* (1978)

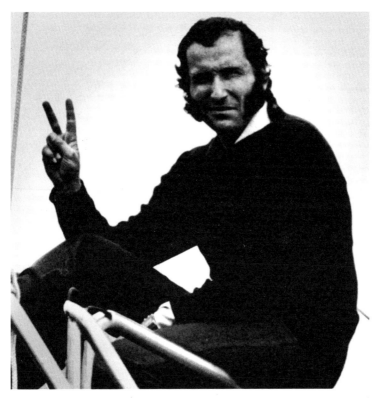

Alain Colas gives a victory sign on board the largest sailing vessel ever to be sailed single handed, Club Mediterranee

Alain Colas was born in Clamercy, near Nevers in Burgundy, on 16 September 1943. Being born in the centre of France, he had no opportunity to learn to sail but he became a keen canoeist on the local rivers and canals. He studied English and French literature at the Sorbonne in Paris and, at the age of 22, left France to go to Australia. His father had shown Alain an advertisement from Sydney University seeking a French lecturer. Alain had no qualifications for such a post but, not properly understanding the language and thinking it merely meant a teaching assistant, applied for the post. Ignoring a letter of refusal, he set off on a freighter for Sydney. Once there Alain used all his powers of persuasion to get the college to accept him. The University eventually relented and appointed him to a French teaching post at St John's College.

In Sydney, Alain took up sailing and discovered a love for it. He crewed on yachts taking part in some of Australia's longest ocean races. In 1968 he shipped as cook on board the yacht *Kahurangui* in that year's Sydney Hobart Race, in which race Eric Tabarly was taking part with his *Pen Duick III*. Colas went on board before the race and met Tabarly for the first time. After the race Colas heard that Tabarly and his crew were proposing to take *Pen Duick III* on a cruise to New Caledonia and he asked if he could come along as cook. Tabarly, after asking who this guy was and not having a cook, agreed. Alain quickly became one of Tabarly's closest disciples and probably the most famous of his many protégées, learning everything he knew from 'the master'.

After this trip, the call of the sea became too great and Colas left his post at the university to join Tabarly for good. He sailed with Tabarly back to France and helped with the building and preparation of the trimaran *Pen Duick IV*, in which Tabarly proposed to enter the 1968 OSTAR.

Colas spent 1968 and 1969 sailing with Tabarly on *Pen Duick III* and *Pen Duick IV*, during which time he learnt his seamanship. In 1969 he was part of the crew of Pen Duick IV when she crossed the Atlantic in a record time of ten and a half days. They then traversed the Panama Canal and sailed up the west coast of North America to Los Angeles. There they entered and won a race from Los Angeles to Honolulu, outstripping all the opposition.

In Honolulu, Tabarly hoisted a large 'for sale' sign on *Pen Duick IV* but finding no buyer went on to Tahiti and then to New Caledonia. Alain had, by now, become enamoured with the trimaran and the Pacific and wrote 'sailing the Pacific is the stuff of which dreams are made.' He set about raising the money to buy *Pen Duick IV* and took a quick trip back to France but with little success. Undaunted, Colas used his Australian savings as a down payment and, with the aid of a bank loan, raised enough to pay Tabarly the 225,000 Francs (about $45,000) that he wanted for the boat. Thus the famous partnership of a man and his boat was formed.

Alain immediately sailed to Tahiti, which to him was close to paradise. There he met Teura who was to become his lifelong friend, companion and ultimately wife, bearing him three children. Teura agreed to sail back to Europe with him. But on the first leg of the voyage from Tahiti to Mauritius, she was too seasick to continue and flew back to France. Colas decided to sail *Pen Duick IV* alone and non-stop back to France via the Cape of Good Hope. He reached La Trinité-sur-Mer in February 1972 after 66 days at sea: then a record for a solo voyage – averaging

150 miles a day over a distance of 10,000 miles.

By the beginning of June, Alain was in Plymouth with *Pen Duick IV* ready for the OSTAR starting on 17 June. He was there along with Tom Follett in *Three Cheers* and Mike McMullen in *Binkie II*. All eyes however were on the huge 128-foot *Vendredi Treize*, owned by film director Claude Lelouch, and to be sailed by Jean Yves Terlain, another of Tabarly's protégées. The boat had been designed by the American designer, Dick Carter, and had the simplest possible rig of just three boomed self-tacking staysails, each on their own mast. Everyone was amazed that one man could handle such a beast but Terlain was convinced he could win the race in a time of under 20 days. No one really realised that Alain was a potential race winner, fully prepared and ready in his strange looking spidery trimaran. It was the largest multihull in the race but looked bruised and battered from its recent voyage from Tahiti.

Light weather predominated for most of the race. Colas reached Newport first in a record time of twenty days, beating *Vendredi Treize*, which arrived a day later in second place. This was the first appearance in Europe of the trimaran *Three Cheers*, which came in fifth in a time of 27 days.

During the race Alain had the almost unheard of experience of crossing tacks with *Vendredi Treize* in mid ocean and overtaking her. He knew then that he would win the race, which he later described as the most beautiful moment of his life. As a result of the ensuing publicity, Alain was able to repay his debts. Now growing in confidence, he was rapidly becoming a favourite of the French media. With his Gallic charm, long black hair and exuberant sideburns he was every inch the sailing rock star. He began to use his infectious smile and personality to good effect in his many TV and press interviews.

On his return to France, Alain announced that for his next project he would become the first person to circumnavigate the world alone in a multihull. Whilst multihulls had sailed around the world before with a crew, it was still not readily accepted that they were safe vessels for a single-handed circumnavigation. The first multihull circumnavigation had actually taken place in 1971, when the English couple, Rosie and Colin Swale with their daughter Eve, had sailed around the world via Cape Horn in a slow and heavy 30-foot Bobcat cruising catamaran called *Anneliese*.

Colas now made some major alterations to *Pen Duick IV*, which he had by now renamed *Manureva*: meaning 'bird of passage' in Tahitian. He said that he had to 'Cape Horn-ize' her, to transform her into a craft capable of sailing safely through the dangerous seas of the roaring forties and furious fifties. He added sponsons to the long thin bows of the three hulls to help prevent them from burying themselves when running fast in large seas. He added a fourth crossbeam near the bows to give added rigidity to the boat's structure. He modified the rig, the self-steering system and the interior, adding radio equipment and distress radio beacons. He had the entire structure of the boat examined using ultrasonic and x-ray scans carried out by the French Atomic Energy Commission. These tests revealed a lot of corrosion to the aluminium structure. This was all repaired. Finally, he repainted the boat midnight blue and put an escape hatch in the bottom so he could get out in the event of a capsize.

Colas raised sponsorship from Radio Television Luxembourg, the drinks company Paul Ricard and the French bank Credit Agricole. Between them they put up enough money to pay for these works. When *Manureva* set off she was probably the best equipped vessel which had ever attempted such a voyage.

Colas and *Manureva* set off from St Malo on 8 September 1973. He had set himself a target to beat the record set by the *Cutty Sark* to reach Sydney in under 80 days. He planned a course to skirt the Canary Islands, Dakar and the Cape Verde Islands, then to cross the equator into the South Atlantic against the south eastern trade winds. Then round the Cape of Good Hope and through the roaring forties across the Indian Ocean and south of Australia to stop at Sydney.

Colas made it to Sydney in 79 days, arriving on 27 November. He had sailed a little over 14,600 miles at an average speed of 7.7 knots. It was a new solo record. On arrival he was met by Teura, his parents and many old friends.

He left for the return half of the voyage on 29 December, the same day as his mentor Eric Tabarly left Sydney in his *Pen Duick VI* on the next leg of the Whitbread Round the World Race which Colas was shadowing.

He had a rough ride across the Southern Ocean and suffered many breakages and gear failures. On 2 February he was met by the British Antarctic survey vessel, the *Endurance*, which escorted *Manureva* through the night as she neared Cape Horn. The next day, in calm conditions, an inflatable put off from the *Endurance* with spare fuel and some supplies.

Much to Colas' disappointment, in almost perfect conditions with calm seas and an azure sky, *Manureva* rounded Cape Horn later that day. He expected, and perhaps longed for, a struggle with storms and high seas. He said later that he felt the good weather had reduced the whole thing to a charade.

Manureva and Colas arrived back in St Malo on 28 March

1974, 90 days out of Sydney. His voyage was a magnificent achievement and he received a hero's welcome.

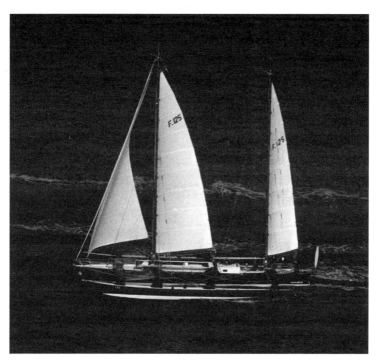

Manureva, with Alain Colas at the helm, at the start of the
1978 Route du Rhum race

After a short pause in France, Colas took *Manureva* to Plymouth for the 1974 Two Handed Round Britain and Ireland Race, which started on 6 July. He was up against fierce competition with the likes of Robin Knox-Johnston in his 70-foot catamaran *British Oxygen*, Phil Weld with his Newick-designed trimaran *Gulf Streamer* and, of course, Mike McMullen with *Three Cheers*.

Colas did not do well in this race and admitted afterwards

that he had underestimated the competition. *Manureva* was grossly overweight as Colas had not had time to unload the heavy radio and other equipment and spare parts he had on board for the circumnavigation. He finished in fourth place, twenty-four hours after the winner. Colas returned to France and began preparations for his next project, which would come to be called his 'magnificent mistake'.

The Royal Western Yacht Club, realising they had a huge, almost uncontrollable, success on their hands, made a number of rule changes for the next OSTAR due to start in 1976. Their first idea was to limit the size of yachts allowed to enter, but agreement could not be reached and, apart from dividing the fleet into three classes, they failed to impose any upper size limit. The rules were published late in 1972 and at first it seemed that the organisers would be swamped by the number of entries. Over 600 people applied.

Colas had in mind something for this race which would startle the world. To make sure he properly understood the rules, Colas telephoned the Royal Western Yacht Club to ask whether he was right and that there really was no upper size limit. Jack Odling-Smee, the race secretary, confirmed this was indeed the case and remarked, somewhat jocularly, that as long as Colas could get his boat into Millbay Dock in Plymouth for the scrutineering it would be all right. At that stage Odling-Smee had absolutely no idea what Alain had in mind and came to regret the remark.

In February 1975, someone sent Odling-Smee a press cutting from *Nice Matin*, a French daily newspaper, announcing plans for a boat to be called *Manureva* (actually it came to be named *Club Mediterranee*) to be sailed by Alain Colas in the 1976 OSTAR. The boat was to be a four masted schooner of an astonishing

236 feet overall length (almost double the length of the largest boat ever to have taken part in any previous OSTAR).

At first the race committee decided to turn down the vessel should such an entry be received and informed Colas of this. Colas then asked to appear before the committee to argue his case. They agreed to see him and Colas told them that the boat was to be fitted with a number of electronic devices to give warnings of ships and icebergs and he emphasised that no sail on the proposed boat was larger than the sails he had handled on his solo circumnavigation in *Manureva*. The committee was swayed by Colas and eventually voted by a majority to allow his entry. They really had no alternative, their own rules not having imposed any upper size limit. The committee received a lot of criticism from the British press and elsewhere for allowing what was considered to be an absurdly large boat to sail across the Atlantic with only one man on board. The UK Department of Transport weighed in, worried about the number of boats allowed to enter, the size of some of these, their skippers' inability to maintain a proper look out and the possibility of damage to other boats if in collision. A normal sized small yacht would come off worse in a collision with a merchant ship or a fishing boat. Not so in the case of *Club Mediterranee*, which could inflict considerable damage. Through all of this Alain was quietly getting on with his plans in France.

Somehow he raised sufficient funds to start work on the boat, which was to be built in the Naval dockyard at Toulon. The massive steel hull, the largest sailing yacht ever to have been built in France, was built upside down to plans drawn up by naval architect Michael Bigoin. The design was wind and tank tested in the French National Aeronautics Research Centre. The boat was to be fitted with state of the art electronics (which were all very primitive by today's standards) and included a satellite positioning system, a computer and fax machines all powered by wind, solar and hydro generators. A closed circuit video system would allow Colas to monitor the sails from an enclosed bridge deck.

Then on 19 May 1975, before he had raised all of the money needed, Colas suffered a serious setback. Whilst attempting to anchor his old trimaran *Manureva* in La Trinité-sur-Mer, his right leg became trapped in the anchor cable whilst it was running out. His right foot was virtually severed at the ankle.

Colas was taken to hospital in Nantes where the doctors doubted if he would ever walk again. They wanted to amputate what was remaining of his foot. Colas refused to allow this. Eventually after a series of some twenty-two operations, many undertaken without anaesthetic at the behest of Colas who wanted to remain alert at all times, Colas recovered and was able to limp around the hospital. Nothing could stop Colas with his project and he continued to manage it from his hospital bed. He drafted in his brother, Jean Francis, who commuted between Nantes and the Toulon shipyard. He sold the rights of his story to the French press to raise more funds.

Even then, all he had was a bare hull and not enough money to buy the masts, sails, engines and equipment. However, his story came to the attention of the Club Mediterranee organisation who agreed to commit two thirds of its advertising budget to the project. This gave Colas enough money to finish the boat.

In July 1975 Colas wrote from his hospital bed to the OSTAR Race Committee saying 'surgeons have done wonders and I shall join the party next June for the race to Newport.' The committee were not so sure and met with Colas in February 1976, accompanied by his doctor who was himself a yachtsman. Colas hobbled into the meeting room and his doctor said afterwards that for all the good the foot did him he might as well have done without it. However, Colas managed to sway the committee, who agreed he could enter provided he undertook an additional single handed qualifying cruise of 1,500 miles between not more than four points in the North Atlantic. Everyone else had to do only a single 500 mile qualifying cruise – Colas had to do that as well. This whole provision angered Colas but he agreed to it, even though it gave him little time, along with all the other preparations needed, before the race in June.

Eventually the monster yacht was launched, fitted out and made ready to sail. Colas undertook the solo 1,500-mile qualifier (and the 500-mile one) and then, with a large crew on board, set sail for Plymouth.

Moored up in Millbay Dock, *Club Mediterranee* dwarfed everything else in sight and was the centre of attention. David Palmer, then news editor of the *Financial Times*, who was also taking part in the OSTAR in his salmon pink Kelsall trimaran *FT*, brilliantly described the atmosphere on board the monster boat:

The boat was alive with women – sensuous French girls with shining faces, pouting mouths and long lissom figures. I went on board one evening to see Colas, and wandered below deck to find a great cavern of a boat with no fittings of any kind – she felt like the inside of an empty cross-Channel car ferry. There was a young man in front of a stove, officially cooking a meal, at this moment in a clinch with his assistant. There were what seemed like two dozen girls sitting next to hammocks strung up between the steel bulkheads. I don't know who they were or what they were doing, but they seemed to belong on board, and as Colas came limping up to them they all

chanted in unison: "Bonsoir Alain," and he, like a feudal baron acknow-ledging the tributes of his retainers replied: "Bonsoir mesdemoiselles."
Back in the wheelhouse, bedlam. A French couple were going at each other hammer and tongs in high-decibel French over which of them was responsi-ble for disciplining their thoroughly undisciplined child.

Colas was, at first, his usual friendly self, limping around the boat with his useless foot, showing off his creation to visiting guests. But all this bonhomie soon disappeared as the pressures on him became too great. The race committee were out of their depth with Colas' monster and drafted in experts from the Royal Navy to look at the boat's computerised navigation and other systems. It was clear that some of these were not allowed by the rules and the committee informed Colas that he would have to disable some of the computer's functions to make them inoperable. This was too much for Colas who, at a bad tempered press confer-ence, bitterly abused the committee not only about this but also about making him undergo the extra qualifying trip.

David Palmer wrote: 'And now here he was in Plymouth, walking on a foot that had no right to be there, about to sail a boat no one wanted to win, knowing that for him to finish sec-ond would be a terrible defeat. Quite suddenly, charming, kind, helpful Alain Colas blew a fuse...This was not to be Colas' year and perhaps he sensed it.'

None of this augured well for the race. On top of this, his old mentor and friend Eric Tabarly in his much travelled *Pen Duick VI* was heavily tipped as the likely winner. Colas' sponsors, who had invested heavily in the project, were expecting him to win and were not pleased at what was going on in Plymouth.

Things did not turn out well for *Club Mediterranee* or for Colas.

The race was run in very heavy weather and the fleet was battered by severe gale after severe gale, with many boats retiring. During the first gale Colas suffered sail and halyard damage but continued. After the second gale he could no longer set the sails to properly balance the boat. He started out with five halyards on each of his four masts but now had only a few left. Colas decided to put into St John's in Newfoundland to reeve new halyards and repair his sails.

Unbeknown to Colas, at the time he turned for land he had been leading Tabarly by some 300 miles and he could have gone on to win.

As a result of this diversion to St John's, Colas arrived in Newport in second place, seven and a half hours behind Tabarly. Worse was to follow. Someone had spotted that Colas had helpers on board *Club Mediterranee* as he left St John's. They hoisted his sails and then disembarked at sea. The race rules clearly prohibited this. They stipulated that people may come on board only when the boat is actually moored or anchored. For this infringement Colas was awarded a penalty of 58 hours (10% of his elapsed time). This dropped his position to fifth.

Clearly 1976 was not Alain's year and was something from which he never really recovered. *Club Mediterranee* was sold and converted into a luxury sailing cruise ship. Renamed *Phocea* she is still sailing today and can accommodate up to 20 passengers in great luxury.

To get back into the mainstream, Colas decided to enter the inaugural Route de Rhum single handed race from St Malo to Guadeloupe, to be held in 1978. This was to be a big, heavily promoted and publicised French jamboree, entered by all the top French 'rock star' sailors. Alain would have liked to have built himself a new boat for this prestigious race but the *Club Mediterranee* experience made sponsors shun him. Colas was not in favour. He abandoned plans for a new boat and got his old well-travelled mount *Manureva* back into commission. He would do the race in her instead.

There were 36 entrants for the Route de Rhum. These included his former sailing companion Olivier de Kersauson and most of the famous names in solo sailing. When Colas arrived at St Malo people commented on the fact that *Manureva* looked worn and tired. She was by now an old boat which had travelled many thousands of miles, including two circumnavigations and several Atlantic crossings. There was visible corrosion in her multiple aluminium cross beams and the aluminium hull plating was battered and bent. This entry was a distinct come down from the hullabaloo surrounding his *Club Mediterranee* days.

The race started from St Malo on 5 November 1978 and the fleet soon disappeared over the horizon. In those days there were no tracking devices and no requirements to report one's position as there are today. Few carried long distance radios and no one knew where the fleet was or who was winning until the boats appeared over the horizon at the finish.

Colas, however, did have his long range radio on board *Manureva* and he regularly reported his position. On 16 November 1978, eleven days out, he sent a radio message saying he was passing the Azores, that everything on board was alright and that he was sailing well. He did not give any detailed position and this turned out to be his last message.

After that nothing further was heard from him and neither his boat, nor his body, nor any wreckage has ever been found.

It is likely that *Manureva* suffered structural damage either from bad weather (or maybe just from corrosion) or as a result of a collision, when she broke up and sank. What must be appreciated is that *Manureva* was very different from today's multihulls which have fully buoyant floats and cross beams. The advantage most often claimed by multihull supporters is that, whilst they can capsize or suffer structural failure, they are unsinkable and will provide a safe rescue platform even when inverted. *Manureva*, however, was not like that. Her floats were designed to be submersible when the boat was hard pressed under sail and her aluminium beams gave no floatation support. Thus if the cross beams broke or a float was holed and the boat capsized she would, in all probability, sink.

Alain Colas will always be remembered for his ill-fated monster but he should really be remembered as a superb seaman who undertook several outstanding voyages, wrote some exceptional books and was an inspiration to a whole generation of young sailors, both in France and elsewhere.

Chapter 6

The Last Voyage and Loss of the Trimaran *Bucks Fizz* and the Loss of her Entire Crew in the Fastnet Race of 1979

When I was preparing my trimaran *Whisky Jack* for the 1979 Azores and Back Race I learnt that a friend of mine, Richard Pendred, who some years before had caught the 'multihull bug,' had recently bought the 38-foot trimaran *Bucks Fizz*. At that time, I was a solicitor practising in London and Richard was the brother-in-law of a good client of mine. *Bucks Fizz* was designed by Dick Newick and was a near but slightly smaller sister ship to his *Three Cheers*. *Bucks Fizz* was also painted bright primrose yellow and shared the same distinctive large turtle deck between the three hulls. She had been built the year before and was new and untried. The first owner and builder of the boat had entered her in some short inshore races but she had never undertaken any longer trips offshore.

Having sailed and raced monohulls for many years, Richard's first venture with multihulls was with an Iroquois catamaran called *Catawampus* which he raced with some success. He then bought a 35-foot Kelsall designed trimaran called *Runaround*. She had been built on the Isle of Mann by Nick Keig and was well known under her original name, *Three Legs of Mann*. She was a very fast boat and in her Nick Keig had won the 35-foot class in the 1974 Round Britain and Ireland Race and was first overall in the 1975 Azores & Back Race. In 1978 Richard sold *Runaround* and bought the larger and faster *Bucks Fizz*. Richard's life was all about racing boats and he was a very competitive sailor.

After arriving back in England from the Azores, I entered *Whisky Jack* for the multihull section of the Fastnet Race which was to start in August of that year. It was the first time that multihulls had been allowed to participate and I was delighted when I found out that Richard was also proposing to take part with his newly acquired *Bucks Fizz*. It would have been a good race for the two yellow trimarans. *Bucks Fizz* was a much faster, but untried, boat while *Whisky Jack*, which had crossed the Atlantic twice, was well-travelled and proven but slower.

The multihull race was fixed to begin after the main fleet had left Cowes and a start was arranged by the Multihull Offshore Racing and Cruising Association (MOCRA) to take place off Yarmouth on the Isle of Wight at four o'clock in the afternoon of the main race start.

A few weeks before the start date for the Fastnet, I withdrew my entry from the race. Looking back on it now I am not really sure why but I began to have bad feelings about the whole thing – a premonition would be too strong a word – but something niggled me about taking *Whisky Jack* out into the Atlantic and the Fastnet rock at that time. To rationalise my decision, I put it about that my partners would not let me take more time off work, having already been absent from the office for eight weeks during the Azores Race earlier that year. My crew, who had been with me to and from the Azores, were clearly very disappointed.

After my withdrawal, I was asked by MOCRA if I would go to Yarmouth and supervise the multihull start. This was to include checking that all entrants complied with the MOCRA safety rules and to see the boats off.

I arrived in Yarmouth on the morning of the start not knowing whether any other boats apart from *Bucks Fizz* would turn up. Soon after midday, whilst the main Fastnet fleet made its way down the Solent then through the narrows at Hurst Fort and out into the English Channel, I spied the unmistakable sight of a yellow trimaran weaving and dancing its way towards us. Whilst waiting for her to arrive I listened to the BBC Radio Shipping Forecast broadcast at two o'clock so I could give the crew the latest weather information. The forecast predicted 'South westerly winds, force four to five increasing to force six to seven for a time.' This was nothing to worry about and pretty well what to expect for the sea areas to which the boats were heading.

Bucks Fizz arrived and picked up a mooring off Yarmouth Pier. I was taken out in the yacht club's launch to be greeted by an ebullient Richard who was in ecstatic form, geared up for what was his first proper race in his new boat. He introduced me to his crew and handed me a crew list, a MOCRA race requirement, with the names and contact details of all on board.

I must admit that I found the boat in a pretty shambolic state with loose gear, food and clothes all over the cabin floor and on the bunks. However, it must be remembered that multihulls, unlike monohulls, do not heel over when at sea and it is not so necessary to store all gear securely. Richard did admit that they had not had time to store things properly. I went through a check list with him to ensure that they had on board flares, life jackets, charts and navigation equipment, anchor and cable, emergency location beacon (EPIRB) and the other rule requirements. Everything seemed in order, although I do recall I was concerned that the life raft was lying loose in the cockpit and that there did

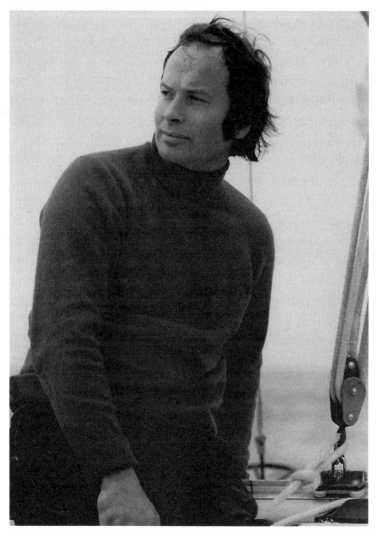

Richard Pendred, owner and skipper of Bucks Fizz

not appear to be any fairleads or bow roller from which to lay out an anchor, which was itself stored on the cabin floor. I do not believe there was any sea anchor. I was also a bit taken aback as it became apparent that the crew did not know each other, nor had they been on the boat before. Apart from Richard, none of them had any experience of sailing multihulls. I did talk to Richard on the foredeck about this whilst out of hearing of the others but Richard, who was all fired-up rearing to go, looked around him and seeing that no other boats had arrived for the start told me he intended to set off and sail after the Fastnet fleet whatever I said, even if he was alone and I refused his entry.

There was nothing I could do to stop him if he decided to go and there was no way for anyone to know what was waiting for them out in the Irish Sea. The forecast gave no hint of a building storm and I considered that *Bucks Fizz* technically complied with the letter of the MOCRA safety regulations.

I said goodbye to the crew and told Richard that we would

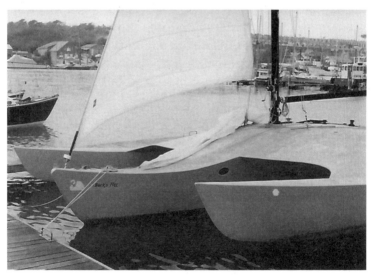

Bucks Fizz

fire a starting gun at four o'clock. The boatman took me ashore. No other multihull arrived, so at four o'clock the gun was fired. *Bucks Fizz* sailed jauntily across the line with all sail set heading west down the Solent in a light south westerly breeze. She looked beautiful in the afternoon sun as she dipped and danced and disappeared through the Hurst narrows. This was the last time anyone on land was to see *Bucks Fizz*. I watched her go with a mixture of anxiety and jealousy. Anxious as to whether they really should be going but also wishing it was me in *Whisky Jack* who was sailing with them.

A few days later I listened to the news coming in from the race with growing apprehension and alarm, as did everyone in the country and around the world. After the start in relatively calm conditions, a large depression, known as low 'Y', formed over the Atlantic during the Saturday of the start and began to develop during the next day, Sunday 12 August. On Monday, this low 'Y' began to intensify and move north eastwards toward the south of Ireland. By Tuesday it was centred over Wexford and the Meteorological Office was receiving reports of gale force winds, with the strongest right over the area where the race fleet was.

The Meteorological Office assessed the maximum wind force as Storm Force 10 on the Beaufort Scale but many race competitors believed the winds reached Violent Storm Force 11 (one Force on the scale below a Hurricane). Over the two days of 13 and 14 August, out of the 306 yachts taking part in the official race 5 were sunk, 100 suffered knock downs and 75 were flipped upside down. 15 sailors died and only 86 boats finished the race. The rest limped into various harbours in Wales, Ireland, Devon and Cornwall.

Rescue efforts began on the evening of 14 August, by which

time the winds had abated to a Force 9 gale. Royal Navy ships, RAF Nimrod jets, helicopters, lifeboats, a Dutch warship and a number of tugs, trawlers and tankers all took part. 125 yachtsmen were picked up.

During the rescue operation there was no mention at first of *Bucks Fizz* but then on 15 August, a fishing boat went to investigate the upturned hull of a yellow trimaran which had been sighted south of the Old Head of Kinsale. They found the boat upside down with no life raft on board and with its centreboard still in the lowered position. The bodies of three crew members were found in the water nearby and the body of the skipper, Richard Pendred, was later found in the yacht's life raft. None were wearing life jackets although three were wearing safety harnesses. The bodies were recovered and landed at Barry in South Wales.

It was not until much later, once crews and boats had returned to land, that reports emerged of *Bucks Fizz* being seen at eight o'clock in the evening on 13 August by two yachts taking part in the race, *Battlecry* and *Condor of Bermuda*. They were both some 45 miles short of the Fastnet rock. Their crews reported the trimaran as moving very fast in 20-25 knots of wind under full sail. At half past three in the morning of Tuesday 14 August, with winds gusting at over 60 knots, the yacht *Pepsi*, lying a-hull having lost her rudder, reported red flares close by. At eight o'clock the next morning her crew saw a capsized yellow trimaran near to them, presumed to be *Bucks Fizz*.

A few days after the bodies had been recovered I received a telephone call from the South Wales Police asking me, as the last person to have been on board *Bucks Fizz* before she set sail, whether I was prepared to go down to Barry to identify some of the bodies which they had found and which had no identification on them. They were believed to have come from the trimaran. I agreed to do this and hoped this would avoid Richard's widow having to go and undertake such a distressing task.

I travelled to South Wales the next day and was able to identify the bodies of Richard and two of his crew. It was a troubling and traumatic experience, the first time I had ever done such a thing and, looking at the bodies laid out in the mortuary, brought home to me that it could easily have been myself and my crew, Julian Mustoe and Roger Hill, lying there instead.

What happened to *Bucks Fizz* is pure speculation but the conclusion of a report carried out by MOCRA into the incident is that *Bucks Fizz* capsized by wave action whilst lying a-hull with no sails set. Whilst I believe it unlikely that *Bucks Fizz* could have survived in those circumstances, a contributory factor to the capsize might have been the fact that her centreboard was in the lowered position when she was found. This lowered centreboard would have prevented the boat from sliding sideways with the waves and may have acted to trip her up whilst the boat was being pushed down the face of a wave. I am sure Richard was aware that it was considered best practice for the centreboard to be raised in these conditions but it may be they were simply caught unawares by the speed with which the wind and seas got up. If the seas then become too large to continue to lie beam on, a sea anchor should have been launched from the bow to attempt to keep the boat's bows facing the oncoming seas.

Battlecry and *Condor* were two fast yachts and they would have been amongst the leaders of the fleet, so *Bucks Fizz* must have sailed very fast to have caught them up and I hope that Richard achieved his aim of rounding the Fastnet Rock before the capsize.

For my part I do not consider that my trimaran *Whisky Jack* would have been any luckier and she would undoubtedly have capsized in those conditions. In this case I too, along with my two crew members, may well have perished.

*

Today there is a Fastnet Race Memorial at Holy Trinity Church in Cowes on the Isle of Wight, on which is listed 19 names, the 15 official race competitors who perished plus the names of Richard Pendred, Olivia Davidson, John Dix and Peter Pickering, the four crew members of *Bucks Fizz*.

In 2003 the islanders of Cape Clear Island in Ireland erected a stone memorial with the names of the 15 official competitors who were lost in the race. Some years later Richard Pendred's son, Guy, who was twelve at the time of his father's death, arranged for the names of the crew of Bucks Fizz to be added to those already engraved on the stone. Guy, his mother and his brother Mark, attended a memorial service in 2015 to remember the victims of the race. Mark was only eight years old at the time of the race.

Guy Pendred has told me that his father was initially very keen to take Guy with him on *Bucks Fizz* for the race (Guy's mother was not at all sure this was a good idea). However, Richard decided against this on the basis that the rules of the official RORC Fastnet race prohibited persons under 16 from taking part. Whilst *Bucks Fizz* was not strictly bound by such rules (the MOCRA regulations contained no such prohibition) Richard thought he should abide by the RORC rules. So Guy stayed ashore.

Chapter 7

The Life, Last Voyage and Loss of Angus Primrose and *Demon Of Hamble* (1980)

Angus Primrose was a larger-than-life character known to virtually everyone in the sailing world. With his untidy grey seaman's beard, a lined lived-in face and fierce piercing eyes he charmed all he met.

Angus came to prominence when, as a young naval architect, he joined up with John Illingworth in 1958 to form the firm of Illingworth and Primrose. This soon became one of the foremost yacht design offices in the United Kingdom, producing many designs for ocean racing and cruising yachts and later the designs for an increasing number of glass reinforced plastic (GRP) production yachts.

Angus's partner John Illingworth was another larger-than-life character. He is often known as the father of the sport of offshore yacht racing. He was a career naval officer who spent the Second World War mainly in the Far East. In 1945 he was stationed in Sydney and proposed the first Australian ocean race from Sydney to Hobart in Tasmania. This race, now held annually in December starting on Boxing Day, has established itself as one of the three pre-eminent ocean races in the world, alongside the Fastnet Race in England and the Newport to Bermuda Race in the USA. Illingworth won the first Sydney to Hobart race in

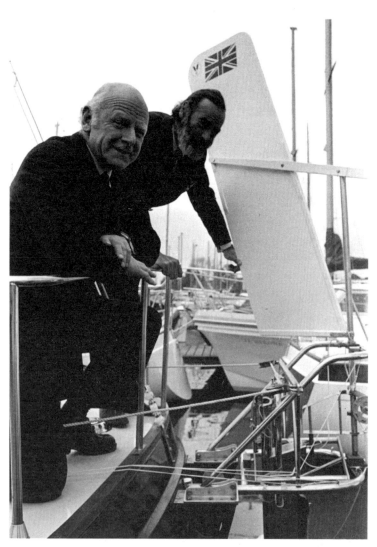

Angus Primrose (with beard) and Blondie Hasler on board Demon Demo,
a Moody 33

his yacht *Rani*. (The only other British yachtsman ever to have won this race was the former Prime Minister Edward Heath in his yacht *Morning Cloud*.)

Illingworth then returned to England and built a series of racing yachts all with the suffix 'Malham', after his birthplace in Yorkshire. His most famous creation was *Myth of Malham*, a controversial design which won many races, including two Fastnet races. The boat was a seminal design from the drawing board of the renowned naval architect Jack Laurent Giles, with much input from Illingworth in relation to the sail plan, rigging and deck layout. She contained many innovations which have now became commonplace in the sport.

In 1950 Illingworth bought a small boatyard in Emsworth in Hampshire called Aeromarine which turned out a number of small ocean racers to his own designs.

Then in 1958, he teamed up with Angus Primrose. The original concept for the firm was for Illingworth to come up with the general idea of a design including layout, rigging and sail plans, leaving Primrose to produce the actual lines of the hull and a builder's specification. Over the next eight years the firm produced a large number of highly successful yachts from the diminutive Top Hat design (basically a mini *Myth of Malham*) to the stately 22-metre *Stormvogel* for a Dutch timber magnate; a co-operative effort between Illingworth and Primrose, Laurent Giles and the Dutch yacht designer Van de Stadt.

Whist at first the lines plans which Primrose produced followed closely to Illingworth's ideas, Primrose soon began to develop his own distinctive designs, shapes and concepts which resulted in many yachts being immediately recognisable as a 'Primrose'.

In the 1960s, the sport of ocean racing was catching on in

France and the firm produced a large number of designs which were built there. A boatyard in Cherbourg started producing one of these, the *Maica* class, on a production line basis.

In 1962 the firm achieved considerable publicity when they were commissioned to produce for Prince Philip a new sail plan and interior layout for the newly acquired royal yacht *Bloodhound*. The next year Primrose produced a striking looking and very fast yacht called *Outlaw* for Sir Max Aitken, then editor of the *Daily Express*. She was beautifully built by Souters boatyard in Cowes which had developed a system of producing cold mould-ed hulls using modern glues and multi-layered thin veneers laid up over a mould, a method which produced a very strong and light hull. *Outlaw* was the biggest boat which had then been built by this method and Souters later turned out many other boats to Primrose's designs.

Then in 1965 Angus was asked to produce the designs for the now famous (or infamous) *Gypsy Moth IV* for Sir Francis Chichester, in which he was to attempt his round-the-world-with-one-stop trip. Angus produced a design which followed the grand old man's precise requirements, including his insistence that the boat did not displace more than nine and a half tons and that no sail was to be bigger than the biggest sail on his old *Gipsy Moth III*, in which Chichester had won the first ever OSTAR. Primrose and Illingworth asked Sir Francis to let them have a free hand on the design so as to produce the best yacht they could but this was refused. The two then reasoned that to do the trip in the time needed (to get to Australia in under 100 days, to beat the times of the old clipper ships), the boat had to have a waterline length of at least 38 feet with long overhangs to give added speed when under way. But the displacement limit on which Sir Francis insisted, together with the need to provide large fuel and water tanks and lots of radio equipment and heavy batteries, meant the boat was built with less ballast than Angus believed was desirable. No wonder then that amongst Sir Francis's grumbles and complaints about the boat was that she was bigger than he had wanted, was too tender and heeled alarmingly, even in a light breeze. After sea trials, Sir Francis grudgingly agreed to allow an extra ton of ballast to be added.

At the launch of the boat, Sir Francis and his financial backer, his cousin Lord Dulverton, had a bad tempered argument with the designers and the builders, Camper and Nicholson, about the cost of the boat. Later Primrose felt very sorry for the yard workmen at Campers who had put everything they could into the building but got nothing but kicks from a cantankerous Sir Francis in his wireless reports and book about the voyage. He pinpointed every minor difficulty in the yacht. A Scottish newspaper reviewing Sir Francis's book reported that the voyage was 'splendid but without charm.' A sentiment with which Angus would surely have agreed.

Primrose never saw eye to eye with the grand old man and their biggest falling out was when Sir Francis reached Australia and sent Angus a telegram stating how he now had 'proper designers design a new keel profile.' Angus's reply was simple: 'Just get on with it. If you've only reached Australia, she's not even run in yet.' According to Angus's son, Dan, what really made his father's blood boil was seeing *Gypsy Moth IV* encased in concrete next to the Cutty Sark in Greenwich.

Several commentators have shared Chichester's criticisms of the boat calling her jinxed, cranky and one of the worst racing yachts ever to have been built. It is reported that, at her launch,

Lady Chichester (as she later became) on seeing the hull react to the wash of a passing ship said "My God, she's a rocker!" Others commented that it would be suicide to take a boat like that out of the harbour.

These are quite unfair descriptions of a yacht which achieved what it did and which, having been dug out of its concrete grave a few years ago, was rebuilt and again sailed round the world, this time fully crewed. She proved to be fast, safe and seaworthy and with few vices. She is still sailing today.

Some years later, one of Angus's colleagues, Angelo Lavranos, who worked with Angus on the design of the boat said it was now time to give the designers credit for Sir Francis's achievements. Angus had to give Chichester the biggest, lightest, fastest boat he could and he did this remarkably well. She had to be light enough to keep moving in light airs and strong enough to cope with the Southern Ocean. It should also be remembered that in 1965 people were not used to light displacement boats. Yachts, especially those considered seaworthy enough to cross oceans, were then in the main small heavy lumbering things with short overhangs and small low aspect rigs. *Gipsy Moth IV* was a new type of experience for most people, but she was exactly what Chichester needed to achieve his objective, even if he did not appreciate that himself.

The whole episode was not a happy experience for the firm. Soon after this John Illingworth retired and went to live in France and Angus continued the business on his own.

One good thing which did come out of this episode was that it led to Angus being commissioned to design several other innovative yachts for other short-handed sailors. Notable amongst these was *Galway Blazer*, built in 1967, and *Ron Glas*, built in 1971, both designed with junk rigs in co-operation with Blondie Hasler.

Galway Blazer was built for ex-navy submariner Bill King for a proposed solo circumnavigation. She was built by Souters in Cowes and exhibited by them at the London Boat Show in 1968. She was a 42-foot-long radical and unusual design with a rounded turtle deck like an elongated egg enclosing the whole hull, with only two small openings near the aft end out of which King could pop his head and from where he could control the sails. The rig was even more radical. The boat carried two unstayed masts from which were hung fully-battened folding Chinese lugsails. This modern version of the old Chinese junk rig had been pioneered by Blondie Hasler on his seminal yacht *Jester* (so named by Hasler as she was 'a bit of a joke'). The advantage of this rig is that the sails could be reefed or lowered by one man just like a domestic window blind, without having to go on deck. The rig was not particularly impressive to windward but performed well with the wind on or aft of the beam, where it should be most of the time on an east about circumnavigation.

King intended to set off on his own in 1968 with no intention of joining a race but his plans were overtaken, much to his irritation, by the announcement in March of that year of the Sunday Times Golden Globe Race, a race in which you were entered by default merely by leaving the United Kingdom before 31 October. At 58 he became the oldest competitor in the race.

In 1971 Primrose produced plans for a yacht commissioned by Jock Mcleod, a Scottish farmer and business partner of Blondie Hasler. He wanted a boat for short-handed racing which he could sail in comfort without the need to get wet (he later boasted that he sailed the Atlantic wearing only carpet slippers). The boat, called *Ron Glas*, was 47-foot-long and was also built by

Souters in Cowes. She had a more conventional coachroof but could be handled by one man through an opening in the cabin top. She too carried a two-masted Chinese junk rig. The boat was a great success and was sailed for many miles by Mcleod, including a Round Britain and Ireland Race and an OSTAR.

However, Primrose's real breakthrough came in 1972 when he was asked to design a 33-foot cruising yacht to be built in GRP. This was to be the first of a series of production GRP yachts to be sold by A H Moody & Sons Ltd., at Swanwick on the Hamble River. Moodys were one of the premier boat builders from the days of wooden boat building and had built up a reputation second to none for the quality of their boats. I had once owned a beautifully built 36-foot One Ton ocean racer built by them in 1964 to a Sparkman & Stevens design, called *Josephine VII*, and exhibited at the 1965 London Earls Court Boat Show. I was twenty two at the time and remember seeing her there and thinking '..mmm, one day...' She was one of the last wooden boats built by Moodys. I bought her in 1985 and kept her for many years, sailing thousands of miles in her.

Moodys, seeing which way the wind was blowing and being aware of the increasing popularity of small boats for family cruising, joined with Marine Projects of Plymouth for them to mould the hulls of a GRP plastic yacht to be marketed by Moodys. The design which Primrose came up with was an immediate success and introduced many of the characteristics found in today's production yachts. Known as the Moody 33, she was modern looking, clean and beamy with high freeboard, a large and roomy central cockpit, a two berth aft cabin, a large saloon and a well-equipped galley. She had a simple masthead sloop rig, a fin keel and skeg rudder and was ideal for family coastal sailing but capable of undertaking ocean voyages. At the time Angus described the boat as his 'block of flats' but she was exactly what buyers wanted and orders poured in.

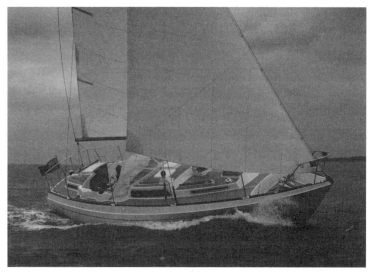

A Moody 33

After this first design, boat followed boat and Moodys launched a whole range of larger and larger GRP yachts, all to Angus's designs and later those of Bill Dixon. In total, during the past 30 years over 4,500 Moody yachts have been produced and sold all over the world.

Following on from this success, Primrose was soon asked to produce designs for other boat builders and a whole series of boats appeared with now well-known names such as Warrior, Challenger, Voyager, North Wind and Seal.

In 1975, to help promote sales of the Moody 33, Primrose entered one in the first two-handed Azores and Back Race (known as the AZAB) which was organised by the Royal Cornwall Yacht Club. The race was from Falmouth to Ponta Delgado in the Azores and back, a distance of 2,500 miles in total, with a crew of only two. He called the boat *Demon Demo*.

The next year, he entered the same boat in the 1976 OSTAR, his first attempt at a solo transatlantic voyage. This was the same ill-fated race in which Mike McMullen and *Three Cheers* disappeared and Sir Francis Chichester had to be rescued. As mentioned earlier, it was a very heavy weather race and many competitors retired as a result of damage. Early on in the race and during the first storm to hit the fleet, *Demon Demo*, sailing with only a heavily reefed headsail, suffered a knockdown and was rolled through 360 degrees. Damage was surprisingly small but she was dis-masted. Angus cut away the rigging and the remains of the mast and rigged a jury mast using a spinnaker pole. With this he sailed over 1,000 miles back to Plymouth arriving safely with no outside help. This was a very fine piece of seamanship.

Maybe this event showed up a weakness of his design and of this type of yacht. Any broad beamed large volume hull is exceptionally stable at small angles of heel but, as the angle increases, so the amount of positive buoyancy decreases until it can reach a point of no return whereupon the boat will capsize. To counter this, a ballast keel is added which increases the righting moment but, in big seas and with a large volume of hull exposed to the wind and sea, such a boat can readily turn right over. A more traditional narrow deep hulled yacht will heel easily at first but is far more stable at large angles of heel and will hardly ever roll right over.

It was soon after Angus's return to England from the 1976 OSTAR that I first contacted and had several discussions with him. The yachting magazine, *Yachting World*, had published the details and lines plan of a proposed design by him for what he described as an 'OSTAR racer', suitable for building by professionals or amateurs, with either a conventional rig or an unstayed junk rig. I was toying at that time with maybe getting involved in such a project and the design I saw appealed to me. I had a number of visits to his design office in Hampshire and he swept me along with his enthusiasm. The matter did not proceed however because the next year I got involved with multihulls, which changed the direction of my sailing. That was when I sailed on a friend's trimaran in the 1978 Round Britain and Ireland Race, in which Angus was also taking part with his repaired Moody 33, now named *Demon*. We had to retire from the race as the trimaran began to fall apart off the west coast of Ireland and Angus had to retire off Lowestoft as he had run out of time.

Angus was back in Plymouth for the 1980 OSTAR with his same Moody 33, now named *Demon of Hamble*. Before the start Angus partied hard and took advantage of his yacht's capacious centre cockpit by keeping it filled with friends and family, the boat floating well below its marks.

This was the first OSTAR which was truly international and was full of the usual controversy involving the French. For the first time all boats were fitted with an ARGOS beacon which transmitted the position of each yacht via satellite, meaning those on shore knew the exact position of each boat, even though other competitors did not. Eric Tabarly had to withdraw as a result of injury. He tried to get the organisers to allow his protégée, Marc Pajot, to take his place, even though Pajot had not carried out a qualifying cruise as required by the rules. Jean-Yves Terlain (another Tabarly acolyte) turned up with a strange looking untried catamaran resembling two waterborne tanks interconnected by a number of large drain pipes (which some people maintained were filled with helium). He had not done any qualifier but told the organisers that whilst he could understand the need for rules he did not see why they should enforce them. (Lloyd Foster, who was central to the organisation of most of these races, remarked that this attitude was familiar to anyone who has ever tried to organise events involving our friends from over 'La Manche'.)

The race was a great success and had a popular winner in the American Phil Weld with his Newick-designed trimaran, *Moxie*. Conditions during the race were generally good and *Moxie* made it to the finish in one hour under 18 days. Angus arrived in just under 31 days, which was a good performance for what was basically a comfortable family cruising boat.

After the post-race celebrations had ended and competitors began to return to their home ports, Angus stayed on in Newport for a few weeks, as he was involved with the unsuccessful British challenge for the America's Cup with the yacht *Lionheart*.

In August, he set off in *Demon of Hamble* to sail her south to Florida, where he intended to sell the boat (and hopefully increase sales of his Moody designs in the USA). He was accompanied by Erica Dobson, a British dental surgeon who came from Redhill in Surrey. All went well with the trip south until they were off the coast of South Carolina. They had taken their time and had sailed over 1,000 miles from Newport. It was now well into autumn, the equinox had passed and gales and storms were frequent in that area at that time of the year. They were also in the area close to the notorious Bermuda Triangle, renowned for many mysterious maritime disasters.

Little is known of exactly what occurred but in the middle of

October they were caught out in a bad storm sweeping the area and *Demon of Hamble* was overwhelmed by the wind and seas. It is presumed that she rolled over (as happened in the 1976 OSTAR) and that the large central cockpit filled with water, weighing the boat down. She may also have lost her mast. Whatever happened, a decision was made to abandon ship and take to the life raft. Angus then launched a raft which inflated itself. Angus got Erica safely into it. Erica said later that Angus then launched another raft which capsized whilst he was trying to get into it and Angus was swept away never to be seen again. Then the yacht went down, leaving Erica on her own in a life raft in the middle of a storm, 180 miles off the coast of South Carolina.

Erica was spotted by a United States navy ship after four days adrift. Erica said later that Angus had sacrificed his life for her.

Angus was then aged 53. He left behind in England his wife, Murlo, and their two children.

His legacy is immense. I doubt if there is a harbour anywhere around the coast of Great Britain, and probably Western Europe, where there is not at least one example of his designs. Bill Dixon, who had been working for Angus for some years took over the business which thrives today. He was only 23 at the time of Angus's death and Moodys remains one of the foremost suppliers of cruising yachts in the United Kingdom.

Chapter 8

The Life and Last Voyage of Rob James on board his Trimaran *Colt Cars GB* (1983)

Rob James was only 36 when he died. Brought up in a large family in southern England (he had three brothers), James soon developed an interest in sailing and was to be found messing about in boats from an early age.

Rob's first involvement in ocean sailing came when he crewed on the newly built *Great Britain II* in the 1977 Whitbread Round the World Race. *Great Britain II* was built for Chay Blyth with a large budget put up by the wealthy tax exile and Britain loving businessman 'Union' Jack Hayward. It was he who had earlier provided the money to rescue Isambard Kingdom Brunel's original *Great Britain*, the first passenger ship in the world to be driven by propellers. With Hayward's money she was returned to her birth place in Bristol; saved from becoming a rotting rusting hulk in the Falkland Islands.

Great Britain II was, at the time, one of the fastest boats in the world but could only achieve sixth place in the race (out of fourteen finishers), probably because she was crewed in the main by a team of paratroopers who were not experienced sailors. It was the first time Chay had skippered a yacht in a competitive race and he was up against some of the world's best.

After the race Rob stuck with Chay and was engaged to skip-

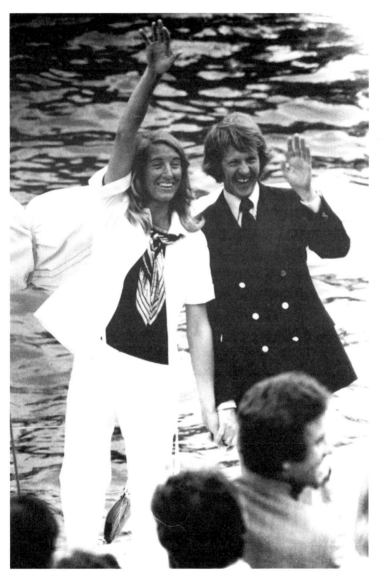

Rob James welcoming his wife, Naomi James, at the completion of her single-handed circumnavigation in 1978

per *Great Britain II* and Chay's other yacht, *British Steel*, on regular trips across the English Channel carrying charter guests. *British Steel* was the yacht which Chay had sailed alone 'the wrong way' round the world in 1970/71.

In 1974 Blyth decided to build a boat in which he could win the 1976 OSTAR. To find the money he went back to the ever generous Jack Hayward who again agreed to put up the money. Blyth was undecided as to what sort of boat he wanted but eventually decided on a multihull as they had done so well in the previous OSTAR. But was it to be two or three hulls? This decision was made after comparing the performance of Mike McMullen in his trimaran, the 46-foot *Three Cheers*, which almost beat Robin Knox-Johnson in his two-hulled 70-foot *British Oxygen* in the 1974 Round Britain Race. It was to be a trimaran.

The boat, to be named *Great Britain III*, was designed by Derek Kelsall, who came up with a monster – 80 feet long and 38 feet wide, weighing in at 13 tons with a massive sloop rig. She was built at Wicormarine in Fareham and Chay Blyth made Rob James his representative to go into the yard to oversee things. The boat, as big as a double tennis court, was fitted out with ten berths, two WCs, a teak lined saloon and a large galley and navigation area – a far cry from today's racing machines. Chay persuaded Dame Vera Lynn to christen the boat on her launch day.

No one had any idea how Blyth was going to handle a boat of this size on his own. She had none of the modern sail handling devices which enable today's sailors to manage huge multihulls alone with ease. Foresails had to be regularly changed by being dragged up from below and hanked on to the forestays with bronze piston hanks. Reliable furling systems had not yet been developed. The huge mainsail descended into a heap on the deck when lowered and had to be bundled up by hand – no stack pack systems or lazyjacks were in use then. The trimaran was full of innovations, some which worked, others which didn't. A single 120 HP engine was to power hydraulic outdrives on each float but this idea never got beyond the design stage.

Rob James' first experience of this monster was when Chay Blyth asked him to take a party of charterers to the Channel Islands. Rob pointed out to Chay that he had never sailed a multihull before and this, his first go, was to be on the biggest one in the world. Just handle it like an ordinary boat was Chay's riposte. Rob got the boat there and back with no auxiliary power and on their return had to sail the boat up the narrow Fareham channel in Portsmouth Harbour to their base at Wicormarine. (I have done this trip often enough in a small 35-foot trimaran and even that was nerve racking enough. How James managed it in *Great Britain III* fills me with admiration.) James also discovered on this trip one of the less pleasant characteristics of multihulls – in the smallest of seas they pitch and jerk in a most alarming manner. Rob skippered a couple of other charters to France in the boat but remained unconverted to the multihull cause.

Blyth next took *Great Britain III* across the Atlantic in a then record time of 10 days from the Cape Verde Islands to the West Indies and sailed her back from New York in another record time of 13 days. After that his luck ran out. While Chay was sailing her alone on his qualifying trip for the OSTAR he collided with a coaster off the Devon coast breaking off one of the floats just forward of the crossbeam. The boat capsized and was towed upside down into Plymouth. She was rebuilt but, unsurprisingly, Chay could not get insurance for the OSTAR. She was sold and converted to chartering and cruising, but never had much luck at that either.

Rob continued his work for Chay and in 1977 he skippered *Great Britain II* in the second Whitbread Round the World Race. This event was a much more professional affair and was dominated by a determined Dutchman in his meticulously prepared *Flyer*. *Great Britain II* came in twelfth out of 15 finishers.

The next year Rob became heavily involved with another Blyth venture, the building of *Great Britain IV*, a smaller but faster replacement for *Great Britain III*. Also designed by Derek Kelsall and once again paid for by the ever-open pocket of Jack Hayward, she was 56 feet long and 38 feet wide with few creature comforts, if any, below. She was built in a great hurry and as light as possible. This resulted in many problems. It meant, amongst other things, (as I later discovered) that you could only put medium tension in the rigging, otherwise the boat bent alarmingly. The whole structure flexed badly in any sort of sea.

Before the Round Britain Race, Rob and Chay took *Great Britain IV* in for the annual Round the Island of Wight race and the Crystal Trophy. This taught them a lot about the boat and showed up more problems. But it also proved to them that they had probably the fastest light weather boat in the world – it was when the wind got up that problems started.

Peter Phillips and I were already moored up in Plymouth in 1978 on our trimaran *Heretic* for the start of the Round Britain Race when Rob and Chay appeared for the scrutineering of their dark red trimaran *Great Britain IV*. She moored up in front of us and behind us was moored *Great Britain II* which Robin Knox-Johnston was proposing to sail in the same race – I well remember hearing Robin saying irritably to Blyth, who was showing him over the boat, "it would obviously be much quicker if you told me what does work, rather than what doesn't."

I went on board *Great Britain IV* and met Rob James for the first time. The boat was certainly impressive and obviously very fast with a towering mast. She made our little 35-foot trimaran look like a minnow. Below she was absolutely dreadful – a long thin coffin-like cabin with no natural light and no ventilation, just a narrow passage with a bench and small galley you could barely squeeze past, then an opening in a bulkhead led to a single narrow berth. Nothing else at all and permeating everything was the overwhelming cloying sweet and sickly smell of the still curing polyester resin used in her construction.

It was then that Rob described to me an alarming feature of the trimaran. When the wind increased and the boat pressed on the lee float, her bows went down rather than rise up. There was too much buoyancy in the back ends of the floats. The ever present lee helm would become uncontrollable and she would suddenly trip round to leeward and try to flip over.

Another problem Rob experienced was that, at times, when going at speed, the helm would become completely unresponsive and no amount of winding on the wheel would make any difference. She just carried on regardless, quite out of control, until the boat slowed. The reason was that, as a wave approached, it lifted the stern until the rudder was completely out of the water. An alarming experience (and something I experienced first-hand a few years later when sailing *Great Britain IV* myself). Modern trimarans have rudders in each of the floats as well as in the main hull to get over this problem.

During the race I met up with *Great Britain IV* again during the stopover in Crosshaven but after that she sped ahead, leaving most of the competitors far behind. Rob described to me their problems on the leg to Crosshaven where they developed a bad leak in one of the floats and sailed the last part of the leg with the float almost submerged and gradually filling with water. They were able to solve the problem before they left for the next leg and thereafter led the fleet for most of the rest of the race.

On the third leg *Great Britain IV* began to fall apart and the crew experienced one breakage after another but somehow managed to keep the thing together, arriving back in Plymouth in the lead just 12 minutes in front of Phil Weld on his new, smart and stylish Newick trimaran *Rogue Wave*. No other boat could keep up with *Great Britain IV*, as long as the wind was light.

Rob's view after the race was that, although the boat did what she was designed for, she was really just a light weather boat and weaknesses in her build were shown up by the numerous breakages. He said it wasn't very clever to go to such extremes in her lightweight construction, when the materials used were not sufficiently strong for the weight. He added that she was basically an unseaworthy boat.

Rob never raced in *Great Britain IV* again but Blyth did enter her later that year in the inaugural Route de Rhum Race from St Malo to Guadeloupe, the same race in which Alain Colas and *Manureva* were lost. Chay suffered from self-steering and other problems from day one and soon retired and headed home to England.

Rob was so impressed by Mike Birch's win in that race, in a tiny 31-foot Newick-designed VAL trimaran, *Olympus Photo*, who beat a long and lean 70-foot monohull, Kriter V, by 90 seconds that Rob bought a sister ship. She was called *Jan of Santa Cruz*, which I remember from the 1978 Round Britain Race when she was raced superbly in the capable hands of Nigel Irens and

Mark Pridie. (Nigel Irens went on to become one of the foremost multihull designers in the world.)

Rob laid up the little trimaran at Wicormarine in Fareham creek for a year and then sailed her to Crosshaven in Southern Ireland to prepare for the 1980 OSTAR. Rob was by then married and living near Crosshaven with his wife Naomi, who, in 1978, had returned to England after her record breaking solo circumnavigation in the 53-foot *Express Crusader* (a boat lent to her by Chay Blyth).

Rob's trimaran which he renamed *Boatfile* (after his sponsors) was one of Dick Newick's VAL class and was basically no more than a 'daysailer' with a central cockpit, which had canvas sides, and a small aft cabin 10 feet long by 2 feet 6 inches wide with only 4 feet of headroom. There was space for a seat, a single burner gas stove and a bunk. In front of the mast was a small sail locker and the boat's small sails could easily be handled from the cockpit. When Dick Newick designed this class he never imagined that anyone would be foolish enough to take one in for a transatlantic race!

In May 1980 James took *Boatfile* to Plymouth for the start of the OSTAR. Naomi was also taking part in *Express Crusader*, now called *Kriter Lady*. Rob and Naomi were the first husband and wife team to compete against each other in an OSTAR. There were to be 88 competitors in this edition of the race, including some very fast new trimarans. Amongst these was the US newspaper publisher Phil Weld in a brand new Newick design which he called *Moxie*. He was the favourite to win and had built the new trimaran because his other one, *Rogue Wave*, was too big for the recently imposed upper size limit.

The OSTAR started on 7 June in good conditions, with

Naomi on *Kriter Lady* towing Rob and *Boatfile* out to the starting line. After the second day *Boatfile* experienced very strong gale force northerly winds which gave Rob some difficult conditions; his little boat did not like it at all. She took a hammering as the floats flexed and slammed into the oncoming seas, sending shivers through the structure. At least Rob could shelter below and simply reach out and alter course on the autopilot without getting out of his bunk. He then had a respite for a few days until another gale hit him on day seven. The next day he had to re-bolt the rear crossbeam where it was coming away from the main hull and he found that water was getting into the starboard float. He had to climb out onto this with a portable pump. He had another gale a few days later which forced him to stop sailing for a while, Rob believing the boat would fall apart if he pressed on.

As he neared the American coast conditions improved, apart from the increasing amounts of fog. On day 19 Rob went below to get some sleep having been on deck staring into the fog for many hours. Just before he dozed off something made him pop his head out of the cabin. He saw a wall of steel a few hundred yards dead ahead. It was an anchored factory ship or a huge trawler and he would have sailed straight into it had he stayed below. He just had time to get out of its way. Day 22 took him over the Nantucket shoals in poor visibility and he crossed the finish line at 0800 on 29 June. He was met by his old steed, *Great Britain II*, who towed him into port.

The first five finishers were all trimarans. *Moxie* was first, arriving in a time of just under 18 days. Rob was sixteenth in 22 days, three days ahead of another Newick VAL. His wife Naomi arrived in 24th place in a time of 25 days, which was a women's record for the race.

Soon after the OSTAR Chay Blyth contacted Rob to say he had found sponsorship to build a new 65-foot trimaran and would Rob like to crew with him in the forthcoming Two Handed Transatlantic Race. This was to be run over the same course as the OSTAR and had only recently been announced by the Royal Western Yacht Club. The race soon became dubbed the TWOSTAR.

This gave Rob a problem as he had already committed himself to sail in this race with Naomi on her *Kriter Lady*, even though the boat, the old *Express Crusader*, was no longer really competitive. But Rob felt Chay's offer was too good to turn down, even though it left Naomi without a crew. This was soon resolved when Naomi teamed up with Laurel Holland, wife of the Irish yacht designer Ron Holland.

After the OSTAR Rob left *Boatfile* in the USA, helped Naomi sail *Kriter Lady* back to England and joined the latest Blyth project. This time the money did not come from Jack Hayward but from Brittany Ferries and the boat was named *Brittany Ferries GB*. She was designed by John Shuttleworth and it was his first independent design, having just left working for Derek Kelsall. She was a very much improved development of *Great Britain IV*, with long tapering high buoyancy floats and three crossbeams, the middle one being under the mast. This produced a very rigid and strong structure and the boat suffered from none of the problems of *Great Britain IV*.

She proved to be a quite different proposition from her forebear. She was very fast (and controllable) and proved to be a good all-rounder in both light and heavy weather. After a trip to Spain and back, the return trip being Chay's and Rob's qualifier for the race, they took the boat to Plymouth for the start. There they were faced with some formidable competition including a handful of impressive new French designs. Robin Knox-Johnston turned up with a new 70-foot catamaran, *Sea Falcon*. Frenchman Loic Caradoc was there with a new 60-foot hydrofoil assisted trimaran called *Royale* with a huge wing mast and there were two very fast looking Walter Green designed 53-foot trimarans, one sailed by Walter himself and one by Mike Birch. Rob and Chay considered Birch to be their main threat. At the bottom end of the fleet was Mark Gatehouse and Michael Holmes in their diminutive Kelsall 30-foot trimaran, *Mark One Tool Hire*. They put up a superb performance.

During the preparations for the TWOSTAR Rob was approached by the builders of the Freedom class of yachts, Fairways Marine, who wanted to build Rob a prototype 70-foot version of one of their cruising yachts to race in the next Whitbread Round the World Race. The yacht was quickly completed and Naomi obtained the agreement of her sponsors, Kriter Wines, to take the new boat into the TWOSTAR, instead of her old and now outdated *Express Crusader / Kriter Lady*. The new boat was named *Kriter Lady II* and had three unstayed masts with three wishbone mainsails and no headsails. It would have been exceedingly good publicity for the builders if Rob had done well in the Whitbread.

In Plymouth before the race *Brittany Ferries GB* and *Kriter Lady II* lay quietly alongside each other in a corner of Millbay Dock. Both were well prepared with everything under control until just four days before the start when Naomi was diagnosed with an ovarian cyst. She went into hospital the next day for an operation. Rob was now faced with not only getting the two boats ready for the race but with making sure Naomi was alright and finding a new skipper for *Kriter Lady II*. With help from all parties, the experienced yachtsman and sailmaker John Oakeley was drafted in to take her place. Naomi's operation was successful.

Four days later the race started in the teeth of a south westerly gale, with more bad weather forecast. *Brittany Ferries GB* made a good start and was soon charging to windward, taking off over the short steep waves, making 16 to 18 knots. This bad weather continued for the first week of the race and decimated the fleet. The French *Royale* was dismasted within an hour of the start, as was another French multihull a few days later. Another lost her rudder. Tabarly's old trimaran *Paul Ricard* retired with a leaking main hull and an Italian trimaran capsized. In all 27 boats retired out of 103 starters and some boats were abandoned. Hardly any boat arrived in Newport undamaged. Several experienced crews said on arrival that conditions were as bad, if not worse, than they had ever experienced in the North Atlantic. *Kriter Lady II* retired with structural problems when they were approaching Newport and they motored to the finish.

During the second week *Brittany Ferries GB* made good progress despite some rigging and sail damage and losing a spinnaker. This wrapped itself around the main hull and both floats taking several hours to bring back on board. Generally, the boat held together well and there was no doubt that her predecessor *Great Britain IV* would never have survived intact in these conditions.

Brittany Ferries GB was first across the finish line in a time of 14 days and 14 hours, a new record. It was a fine performance in a well put together boat in some appalling weather. They were 140 miles ahead of the second boat to arrive, Marc Pajot in *Elf Aquitaine*. There were some amazing performances amongst the smaller boats, including that of *Mark One Tool Hire*, the tiny

30-foot trimaran of Mark Gatehouse, which arrived in only 22 days to win their class. Mark and his crew had sailed virtually the whole way treating the boat like a dinghy wearing wet suits. Another good performance was that of Philip Walwyn and his wife, who arrived after 18 days in fifteenth place in their 45-foot cruising catamaran *Skyjack* (see Chapter 11).

This race was the last which Rob sailed with Chay and they went their separate ways. Chay never repeated the successes he had enjoyed with Rob, who was undoubtedly the best and most competitive sailor of the two.

As soon as Naomi and *Kriter Lady II* arrived in Newport, she and Rob prepared the boat for the return journey to England. The trip was to be crew training for the Whitbread Round the World Race, which was due to start two months later. With a full crew, they put up a very fast time of 13 and a half days, a good time for what was basically a cruising monohull and they nearly beat Blyth in *Brittany Ferries GB* who had left Newport on the same day.

When approaching England at the end of the voyage, Rob was told on a radio link call that Fairways Marine, the owner of their boat, had gone bankrupt. They headed for Dartmouth to work out their legal position. Upon going ashore Rob read in a newspaper of the failure of the company, that *Kriter Lady II* was its only asset and wouldn't Mr James get a rude surprise when he landed in England.

Within hours a writ was fixed to one of the boat's masts. In an attempt to salvage something out of the mess, Rob looked around for someone to buy the yacht so they could continue with the Whitbread. Rob quickly obtained the agreement of Michael Orr, the boss of the Colt Car Company, importers of Mitsubishi cars into the UK, who made a generous offer to the Receiver to buy *Kriter Lady II*. To everyone's surprise this was turned down and that was the end of Rob's Whitbread.

Rob's crew joined Blyth for the race on the old *Great Britain II* and Naomi and Rob cast around as to what to do next. Within a few days they had their next venture sewn up. The same Michael Orr of Colt Cars had agreed to build Rob a 60-foot trimaran to take part in the next Round Britain Race and then to race in the Route de Rhum, both to be held in 1982. Rob decided to co-design the boat with his neighbour in Ireland, the well-respected designer Ron Holland, even though Holland had never designed a multihull before. Ron was the husband of Laurel, who had sailed in the TWOSTAR on board *Kriter Lady II*.

The boat which came off Holland's drawing board was fairly conventional and was built in double quick time by a specialist firm in Cowes, SP Composites, who used what were then very novel materials. The hulls had a Nomex core, instead of the more usual foam or balsa, and they used a mixture of carbon and Kevlar for the cloth. There were some initial problems with the design, particularly the fact that the boat floated bows down and this defect was never properly solved.

She was launched on 7 May 1982 and named *Colt Cars GB*. The next day Rob and Naomi set off on their 200 mile qualifying trip with just over 24 hours to the deadline. Despite periods of calm, they managed to complete the trip in time. After working the boat up, sailing daily from Cowes, they set off at the end of June for Plymouth and the Round Britain Race, where they met the competition they would be up against. First amongst these was Rob's old shipmate Chay Blyth back with *Brittany Ferries GB*, looking threatening with a lengthened mast and a sail

141

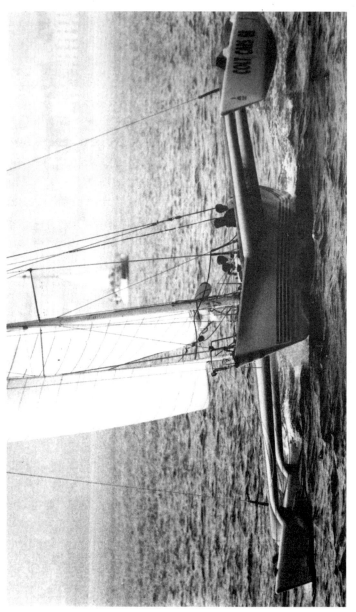

Colt Cars GB in 1983

area increased from 2,000 to 2,500 square feet. Amongst the fleet were some new and very fast trimarans, including Mark Gatehouse with the extremely photogenic *Exmouth Challenge*. My old colleague Peter Phillips, the sailing policeman from Exeter, was there with his new *Livery Dole* (a Shuttleworth design and a smaller version of *Brittany Ferries GB*) and the ever-present Robin Knox-Johnston in his large 70-foot catamaran *Sea Falcon*. Lower down the fleet were two new impressive designs from the up and coming designer Nigel Irens, a handful of new Newick designs and a trimaran called *Twiggy* which had sailed all the way from Australia just to take part in the race. There was also my own small 30-foot trimaran *Applejack* being sailed by my friends Julian Mustoe and Andrew Williams. Philip Walwyn and his wife were back in their well proven catamaran *Skyjack*, newly arrived from the West Indies. All in all, it was the most impressive and competitive fleet that had yet assembled for this race. There were to be 85 starters of which 69 would finish.

The media gave much publicity to the supposed rivalry between Blyth and James. In response to questions such as who will come second and who is your biggest competitor, they each replied "*Exmouth Challenge*", refusing to rise to the bait of naming each other.

The forecast for the start on 6 July was for south westerly winds veering north east, force 4 to 5, maybe increasing to gale force 8 later. This meant a windward beat all the way to Crosshaven and competitors must have had in mind the Fastnet storm of 1979, which started with a similar forecast.

Colt Cars GB started well and had a two-minute lead over Chay's boat at the Eddystone lighthouse. After that and despite the forecast, the wind continued to drop and *Colt Cars GB* quickly ate up the 200 miles to Crosshaven, carrying a spinnaker for much of the way. She was the first to arrive after 22 hours and 4 minutes, beating *Brittany Ferries GB* by 20 minutes.

Exactly 48 hours later, at 9 o'clock in the morning, *Colt Cars GB* crossed the start line for the next leg to Castlebay in the Outer Hebrides, a distance of 460 miles. There was virtually no wind and they sat becalmed for half an hour, losing all their time advantage over Blyth. Eventually a light breeze came up from the south east and they began to move away in poor visibility. That evening they drifted past the Fastnet rock and were still near it five hours later. Eventually, as it always does, some wind appeared, this time from the north, and it quickly increased to a force 6 and *Colt Cars GB* began to pitch badly slamming into a confused sea. Naomi was very seasick. The course was now a dead beat to windward and they began to cross tacks with *Brittany Ferries GB*. Two other multihulls were keeping pace with them further away.

At dawn on the third day they were able to bear away for a straight run to Castlebay. This gave them some hair raising sailing as they charged at 18 to 20 knots into the oncoming seas which hit the crossbeams sending sheets of green water over the deck and at the helmsman. This pounding led to the fairings in front of the box section beams breaking away, resulting in the boat nearly stopping with a shuddering crash each time the square front of the beam hit an oncoming sea. This put a huge strain on the rig and Rob was forced to slow down fearing a dismasting; this allowed some other boats to get ahead. *Colt Cars GB* arrived in Castlebay in third place, 90 minutes behind *Exmouth Challenge* and 30 minutes behind Chay Blyth. During this leg the headboard at the top of the mainsail on *Colt Cars GB* had begun

144

to disintegrate and their sponsors, Colt Cars, obligingly flew in the necessary spare parts by helicopter, so Rob could repair the sail.

The next leg was to Lerwick in the Shetlands and the three leading boats made fast passages out into the Atlantic heading for St Kilda in 25 knots of wind. Once past St Kilda the course was dead downwind and on *Colt Cars GB* they hoisted a large spinnaker. This gave them the worst moment of the race. Rob was at the helm, the boat making 20 knots with spray flying everywhere, when a particularly large wave picked up the trimaran. Rob lost control as she shot down the face of the wave. The lee float dug in. The boat broached ending up stopped and lying beam on to a 30-knot wind with a full main and spinnaker driving the lee float completely under. Rob released the spinnaker sheet and Naomi tried unsuccessfully to get the sail down. Luckily the next wave knocked the boat off the wind, the spinnaker filled and the boat shot off like a rocket. They had been right on the verge of capsizing completely.

They continued on with their speed wavering around 23 to 24 knots, swooping down the waves with the sort of power which quite unnerved Naomi. They nearly capsized again as they gybed to lay a course to Muckle Flugga, the most northerly point of the Shetland Islands. This time a wave hit them at the wrong moment and they lost control, the boat spinning through 180 degrees ending up facing upwind with all sails and sheets flaying in the wind and the mast shaking violently. The boat started to move fast backwards (something trimarans are very good at) and the crew eventually managed to pay her head off. The boat pivoted around on one float, accelerating like a racing car with the other float high in the air. Rob was convinced that the main hull came clear of the water before the hulls smacked back down onto the water. Rob later remarked about the incredible effect a fast multihull has on the apparent wind. Go downwind at 15 to 20 knots and the wind over the deck is only a light 10 knots or so. Turn upwind and you find yourself in 35 knots of wind – a near gale – with full sail set.

The charge continued with one more near capsize before they rounded the headland and turned south. A vicious squall hit them as they neared the finish line, once again submerging the lee float. They crossed the line with the speedometer hard against the 30-knot stop. They finished second, two hours behind *Brittany Ferries GB*. *Exmouth Challenge* came in over two hours later.

For the next leg to Lowestoft they were blessed with a steady westerly wind on the beam and they put in a series of long reaches making 12 or 13 knots; the only problem they experienced was a recurring difficulty in lowering the fully battened mainsail. They finished this leg only 19 minutes behind Chay.

The final leg to Plymouth started in another calm with Chay and Rob drifting helplessly around the start line in a strong tide. Rob anchored whilst Blyth drifted down tide and thereby *Colt Cars GB* took the lead. After four hours a small breeze came in and *Colt Cars GB* set off first, but *Brittany Ferries GB* soon overtook them. Conditions were light and fluky across the Thames Estuary, past the Goodwin Sands and Dover. After that *Colt Cars GB* picked up a good wind and shot off past Dungeness making 16 knots. In a fluky wind they came up on *Brittany Ferries GB* and, by dint of some good sailing from Rob, they gradually overhauled her and covered her all the way home. Rob led his boat into Plymouth by forty-three minutes. *Exmouth Challenge* came in third, one hour later.

Asked at the end whether she had enjoyed the race, Naomi said she had not and that she intended to retire from competitive racing whilst she was ahead. She said it was too hard, mentally and physically, and the way the boats had to be driven was beyond her strength and skill.

This was to be the last race which Rob James completed. He started the Route de Rhum from St Malo later that same year but had to abandon the race as a result of damage to the trimaran.

In March 1983 Rob, with a full crew, was sailing *Colt Cars GB* from Cowes to Salcombe in Devon, where the boat was to be lifted out of the water to undergo a full refit. There were five people on board and, as they were lowering the sails in preparation for entering harbour, Rob James slipped and fell into the netting strung between the main hull and the floats. A rope holding up the netting broke, the netting collapsed and Rob fell through it into the sea. He was not wearing a life jacket or a safety harness. It was said later that Rob did not panic and was still talking to his crew members as he began to drift away. Crew member Geoff Houlgrave, who was asleep at the time of the accident, was awakened and dived in to attempt to rescue Rob. Another crew member tried to turn the boat, which had no engine, so as to get nearer to the people in the water. Geoff managed to make contact with Rob, grabbed him several times but was unable to hold on to him. Geoff had a life line attached to the boat and was hauled back on board with great difficulty and later had to be treated for exhaustion and hypothermia. Rob's body was recovered by the Salcombe lifeboat and taken ashore. He was dead by the time he was found.

The irony of this whole episode was that, having sailed three times round the world and sailing thousands of miles each year, Rob simply took a step backwards, a rope broke and he lost his life. The rope which broke and the netting which it supported were all going to be replaced as part of the forthcoming refit.

Two weeks later Naomi gave birth to her and Rob's first and only child.

Geoff Houlgrave, who tried to rescue Rob, sailed *Colt Cars GB* in the 1984 OSTAR. Nine days into the race on 11 June her mast came down damaging the starboard float. He abandoned the boat in mid-Atlantic and was taken on board a rescuing ship.

The trimaran was later salvaged and recovered by Don Wood. He repaired the damage, rebuilt the starboard float, changed her name to *RedStar / NightStar* and entered the 1986 Round Britain Race, sailing with sailmaker Butch Dalrymple-Smith. It was a heavy weather race and *RedStar / NightStar* suffered more than her fair share of damage. They hit an unlit buoy leaving Crosshaven, damaging the bow of the port float which Don proceeded to repair underway. They finished in fifth place, behind Robin Knox-Johnston in his catamaran (now called *British Airways I*) and Mark Gatehouse in his old *Exmouth Challenge*, now renamed *Marlow Ropes*. (The various changes of name as sponsors changed from race to race was beginning to become very confusing.)

The last race in which Rob and Naomi's trimaran took part was the 1988 OSTAR, no longer sponsored by The Observer but now by Carlsberg. She was sailed by our old friend Chay Blyth; the boat now named *NCR*. However, it was never a serious entry as Blyth had recently fallen off a horse and broken a leg. He was hobbling about on crutches days before the start.

Chay retired three days after the start returning to Plymouth and bizarrely informing the media that the whole thing should be stopped as it was all too dangerous. These remarks were a bit ironic coming from someone who had almost single-handedly invented the idea of dangerous solo voyaging in the first place.

After that I lost touch with Rob's trimaran but no doubt she disappeared somewhere into the burgeoning French multihull fleet, racing under different names until she broke up, sank or was abandoned in the midst of an ocean somewhere.

Colt Cars GB was not a lucky boat.

As for Naomi, she continued to live alone in the small cottage at the entrance to Cork harbour in Ireland, which was the house she and Rob found together after her record-breaking round the world voyage. Their daughter is now 33 and studied psychology at Trinity College, Dublin. In 2006 Naomi completed a Ph.D. thesis on Ludwig Wittgenstein, the German-British philosopher and she now lives in her native New Zealand.

Chapter 9

The Life, Loves and Last Voyages of Peter Tangvald on board *L'Artemis* (1991) and his Son Thomas on board *Oasis* (2014)

In 1959 I was a sixteen-year-old school boy, infatuated with all things to do with the sea, spending as much time as I could during the holidays on board my father's old sailing boat, *Sophie*. She was a ramshackle 35-foot Falmouth Quay Punt built in 1892, moored in the small yacht harbour at Birdham Pool near the top of Chichester Harbour in Sussex. There, I and my sister spent happy days, messing about in boats with the other children off the yachts and with those who lived in houses overlooking the harbour. These included Philip Walwyn and his two sisters (see Chapter 11).

Moored near to us was a smart 35-foot wooden cutter called *Dorothea*. She was well cared for by a distinguished looking naval man, Captain Taylor. The boat was a design from the board of Dr Harrison Butler, then a well-known amateur yacht designer who, over many years, produced a succession of small sensible and seamanlike cruising yachts. *Dorothea* had been built at Whitstable in Kent in 1934 and had the typical Harrison Butler sheerline with a bluff bow and a transom hung rudder. To my ignorant eye she looked extremely seaworthy and was the type of boat I dreamed of owning and sailing away in.

One day, to my surprise, I saw seated in the cockpit of *Dorothea* not the grey haired naval captain but a tanned, handsome young man with short cropped blonde hair and Scandinavian looks. "What are you doing on that boat?" I shouted at him somewhat rudely.

He looked up, gave me a broad smile and said, "I have just bought her. Come on board and have a look."

I did so and thus started an intense and brief friendship with Peter Tangvald. He explained that he had just returned to England to buy a new boat. He had sold his last one in California having sailed her across the Atlantic and through the Panama Canal. That first day he told me all about his voyage and his race across the Atlantic, he in his yacht *Windflower* against Edward Allcard in *Sea Wanderer*. I pricked up my ears at this as Allcard was already a hero of mine and I had avidly devoured his two books *Single Handed Passage* and *Temptress Returns*. Allcard was the first man to sail the Atlantic singlehanded both ways, from England to America and then back to England.

The next day Tangvald asked me if I would be interested in helping him get the boat ready for his planned trip around the world. Being by then a little 'star struck', I could think of nothing I would rather do and said that I would love to. What appealed to me most was that Peter treated me as an adult, which was a rare thing for grown-ups to do in those days. For the next few weeks I worked on *Dorothea*, where I learnt much about preparing a ship for a long voyage. Tangvald simplified everything. He took out the engine, removed the cockpit and built a flush deck where it had been, reinforced the rigging and changed the layout below. He threw out the toilet, preferring to use a bucket, blocked up all underwater seacocks and openings and converted the empty space below where the cockpit and engine had been into a large storage area.

Tangvald told me that he had signed up a very pretty 22-year-old girl to accompany him on his trip. By that time my 18-year-old teenage sister, Olivia, had fallen head over heels in love with Peter (something teenage girls did with regularity throughout the whole of his life) and, had Olivia been a few years older, I am sure she would have fought tooth and nail to have taken that girl's place. But none of that was to be.

I remember the day when an elegant and smartly-dressed lady arrived on the quay and, smiling, said to Peter, "May I come on board, dear?" This was Lillemor, his third wife, who had decided she would join him. Peter, with a great deal of regret, had to break this sad turn of events to his prospective crew. My sister smirked when told the news.

Soon after that they set off to Brixham to complete their preparations for what turned out to be a three-year circumnavigation.

Lillemor did not last beyond Vigo in Spain. She jumped ship after a rough crossing of the Bay of Biscay. She headed home to Norway on a steamship, standing on the deck waving goodbye to Peter as it left. Peter remarked ruefully in his book *Sea Gypsy* that his first wife had waved goodbye through an aeroplane window in Burbank, California. His second from the dirty window of an express train in Los Angeles.

Peter decided to carry on alone, made his way across the Atlantic via the Canaries and then spent some time in the Caribbean. In St Lucia he met an 18-year-old girl with 'almond-shaped eyes and rolling hips' and small golden earrings in both ears. She was called Bjula and claimed to be the daughter of a voodoo sorceress. Before agreeing to sleep with Peter she insisted on piercing his ear, using one of his rusty sail-making needles, and inserting one of her gold earrings in the hole. She then told Peter that with her ring her blood had now got into his and he would die if he ever took the ring out.

Sometime later in Martinique, Peter met a French gym teacher called Simonne who agreed to join him for his trip across the Pacific. Peter said a sad goodbye to Bjula and Simonne remained with him for the rest of his circumnavigation. She later became his fourth wife.

They passed through the Panama Canal and visited the Galapagos Islands, the Marquesas and Tahiti. There, Peter's film star looks got him a speaking part in the making of the film of the *The Mutiny on the Bounty*, starring Marlon Brando and Trevor Howard. Continuing westward they passed through the Torres Strait, crossed the Indian Ocean and stopped at Aden before traversing the Suez Canal. They crossed the Mediterranean and overwintered in Cannes in the south of France. The next year they sailed for England ending up back at Birdham Pool, from where Peter had started three years earlier.

*

Peter's early life involved a succession of failures with a few minor successes and he always suffered from ill health. He left school early, joined the Norwegian Coast Guard, was drafted by the Norwegian Air Force and then trained as a tool and die maker. In 1945, when Peter was 21, he married an 18-year-old school friend and they moved to the USA, where he set up in business as tool and die makers with his father. In America he was divorced twice and re-married twice. Then in 1956 he married Lillemor, an old flame from Norway. Bankruptcy (twice) followed. To

153

make some money he cooked up a plan to travel to England, buy a cheap boat and sail it back to California to sell at a profit.

In 1957 he and Lillemor left for England where, at West Mersea in Essex, Tangvald bought a 45-foot-long yawl called *Windflower*. Lillemor intended to sail with Peter but she left him in Dover after a rough crossing of the Thames Estuary. She returned to Norway.

Peter set off alone calling in at Las Palmas in the Canary Islands where he met Edward Allcard, another lone wanderer on a circumnavigation in his yacht *Sea Wanderer*. The two became good friends and agreed to race each other across the Atlantic to English Harbour in Antigua. The prize was to be one US dollar.

The two boats set off on 20 November 1957. Peter arrived first, thirty days and nineteen hours out of Las Palmas. Allcard arrived a further two days behind. The dollar bill Peter won was signed, framed and mounted on the bulkhead of Peter's cabin as a memory of the first east-to-west transatlantic singlehanded race.

Peter left Allcard in Antigua and sailed on westward. He traversed the Panama Canal and sailed up America's Pacific coast to San Francisco where, in 1958, he sold *Windflower* at a good profit. The next year he returned to England and bought *Dorothea* in Birdham Pool. That was the year I met him and from where he sailed *Dorothea* around the world, arriving back in England in 1963 with Simonne on board.

Peter and Simonne spent a short time in England, enough only for Tangvald to get his book *Sea Gypsy* to the publishers. They then sailed south to the Mediterranean, where they spent a year in Cannes. Peter began to study naval architecture and Simonne found work in a school not far from the port.

Peter had long held a dream of building his ideal cruising boat to his own design. They decided to achieve this by sailing to French Guiana in South America, where supplies of suitable timber were cheap and plentiful and where Simonne could hopefully get a transfer from her job in Cannes. However, just before their planned departure date, Peter suffered a serious heart attack and, after a spell in hospital, was sent to a rehabilitation centre. He was told he might not have long to live. After several months Peter had had enough of his treatment, discharged himself and, still very weak, set off with Simonne to sail to South America. This was in the middle of 1965 and they stopped in Gibraltar where, with Peter barely able to get ashore, the couple were married. They called in at the Canary Islands and arrived at Cayenne in French Guiana at the end of the year. He was now fully recovered but suffered from recurring heart problems for the rest of his life.

Peter rented a house in Cayenne and next to it built a large shed, 60-foot-long by 40-foot-wide, where he would build his boat. She was to be a traditional wooden 50-footer to his own design to be called *L'Artemis de Pytheas*. She was a shallow beamy vessel with a centreboard, a schooner bow and a cut off counter stern with a long low traditional coachroof pierced by small round portholes. She was built without an engine and one was never installed. Peter built the hull upside down and on completion, entirely on his own, turned it over using only ropes and tackles. Over the years Peter experimented with various mast and sail arrangements. The boat started out as a yawl, was then converted to a schooner and finally to a cutter, first without and then with a main boom.

In 1967, before work started on the new boat, Peter decided to sell his faithful *Dorothea* and started out alone for Fort Lauderdale in Florida. One night *Dorothea* hit some wreckage and was holed below the waterline. She sank rapidly some 55 miles east of an island in the West Indies. Peter survived by covering these miles in a 7-foot plywood dinghy, helped along by a favourable easterly trade wind.

Building of the new boat began on Peter's return and she was finally made ready for sea in 1973. During this period Peter had an affair with an 18-year-old schoolgirl called Lydia, who he had first met some years previously in Martinique. Simonne taught Lydia gym at her school and did not believe the affair would last for long. When Lydia's father declared he wanted to leave Martinique and take Lydia away the very year she was due to take her Baccalaureate, the good Simonne offered to take Lydia into their home until she had taken her exams. A few weeks later she found Peter and Lydia in bed together. Simonne had had enough, sought a transfer back to France and left. Lydia stayed on in the house and Simonne and Peter were divorced.

In 1974 Peter, with Lydia on board, sailed *L'Artemis* to Martinique and then on to St. Barts where they stopped long enough for Peter to make a new main mast. From there they headed non-stop to the Mediterranean and France arriving late in the year. They tied up in Port Grimaud where Peter had been lent a mooring for the winter. Unable to find any work locally they decided to leave *L'Artemis* where she was and try their luck in Paris. The winter in Paris was a hard and difficult time for them both. Rents were high and they could only afford a squalid single room with a communal toilet shared with some twenty other tenants. Lydia found poorly paid work in an office and Peter tried his hand at photography without much success. In the spring they left for the south, with much relief and no regrets.

Back on board *L'Artemis*, Peter set about preparing her for a voyage to the Indian Ocean. Before they were ready to leave, Peter was persuaded to take on a job to go to Taiwan to supervise the construction of a number of 52-foot yachts to a French design. To get to China he decided he would sail there in *L'Artemis*. Unfortunately, arrangements with the Chinese dragged on until very late in the year and it was not until January 1976 that he and Lydia were able to leave. Lydia was by then five months pregnant.

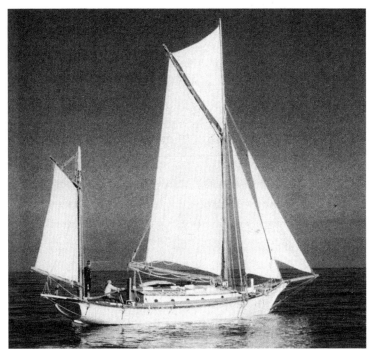

*L'Artemis de Pytheas as she was rigged in 1976
with Peter and Lydia Tangvald at the helm*

The Mediterranean can be ugly at that time of year and so it proved. After passing Malta they ran into some bad storms in which Lydia was violently seasick. They reached Port Said on 23 January and, having no engine, Peter was forced to have *L'Artemis* towed through the Suez Canal. He was not allowed to sail through. They then passed quickly down the Red Sea with a strong following north wind. They stopped in Djibouti, which was still French in those days, and then headed out into the Indian Ocean, eventually arriving in Sri Lanka.

They had planned to have the baby there but one look at the filthy hospital soon disabused them of this idea. With Lydia heavily pregnant, they set sail for Malaysia where they hoped they would find things better. Lydia was not concerned that the baby might arrive before they reached land as she herself had been born at sea. When *L'Artemis* was just south of the Bay of Bengal and still west of the Malacca Strait, Lydia felt the first pains. Two days later she gave birth to a boy, who they named Thomas. It took a further two weeks to reach Singapore where Peter was overwhelmed by the paperwork necessary to gain entry, especially in the case of the baby for whom he had no papers whatsoever. He narrowly avoided being imprisoned and having his boat confiscated for foolishly importing their firearm. They avoided the discovery of it during a Customs search by Lydia lying barely clothed on her bunk and refusing to get up. The gun was underneath the mattress. They hated Singapore which to them was like a police state. They soon set sail, this time for Hong Kong, which they liked. Then they sailed for Taiwan where they remained for two years whilst Peter worked at the shipyard which was building the yachts. They were forced to live ashore to avoid the stench in the harbour, which was really no more than an open sewer.

By the spring of 1978, Peter had fulfilled his contract and he and Lydia had had enough of China. On 10 April they set sail for the open sea, revelling in the sense of escape as the sewer brown waters of Taiwan changed into clear blue ocean sea. Thomas was now two years old. They had no exact destination but just wanted to get away from China. Peter studied his charts and fixed on the Philippines with its hundreds of anchorages and islands. As they departed he wrote 'towards Manila' in his log as their destination.

For nearly a year Peter, Lydia, Thomas and *L'Artemis* wandered through many of the islands, ports and harbours of the Philippines, some good and some very bad. They felt unsafe during their entire stay. In one crowded harbour their boat was badly damaged when a local fishing boat rammed it. Before they could make any repairs, or receive any compensation, they were chased out by threats of violence if they stayed – some of these from the port Captain himself. Peter disliked the corruption and anti-western attitudes of the locals, who preyed on visiting yachtsmen, considering them a nuisance. Lydia was attacked and robbed whilst shopping ashore.

Finally, they moved on to the island of Cebu where they found a safe refuge in a sheltered lagoon; there they recovered and Peter repaired the damage to *L'Artemis*. They were now keen to get back to 'civilisation' and decided to head for Brunei and wait there for the monsoon to turn so as to blow them to Hong Kong. The easiest route to Brunei was via the Sula Sea, which route Peter took despite his knowing of its very bad reputation for pirate attacks.

They sailed on 14 February 1979 and six days later Peter

wrote in his log: 'This morning was boarded by wooden motor-boat and they shot Lydia and killed her. I still can't understand it has happened. Thomas is OK, but cries for his mother and I don't know what to make him eat.'

What happened was that, after they had passed Bancoran Island, they saw a boat very close by following them and steering toward them. Lydia suggested getting their gun and firing a warning shot. Peter told her it was too late for that as the boat was nearly alongside. Lydia went below leaving Peter at the tiller. Then to his dismay he saw Lydia come out of the forehatch with his gun. She fired a shot over the boat which was only a couple of feet away. The reaction was immediate – a shot was fired at her from inside the deckhouse of the other boat. Lydia fell into the sea, staining the water red with her blood. The man who fired the shot came outside and pointed his gun at Peter. This man, however, never fired but hesitated and lowered his gun.

Peter later wrote in his log: 'Only then was I aware of Thomas who was clinging to my leg looking at the strange boat. It must have been the sight of that beautiful little boy with blond hair clinging to his father which softened the man so that he could no longer shoot.'

Two men from the boat climbed on board *L'Artemis* and went below. They came up with all the money they could find, only some 100 US dollars, picked up Peter's gun and jumped back onto the vessel which sheared off and disappeared to the south. The boat was about 50-foot-long, old and dirty but with a smooth and silent engine. Some 12 men were on board.

Somehow Peter managed to continue sailing despite deep feelings of utter despair, guilt and regret. Thomas developed a bad fever and became very ill. They had 150 miles to go to

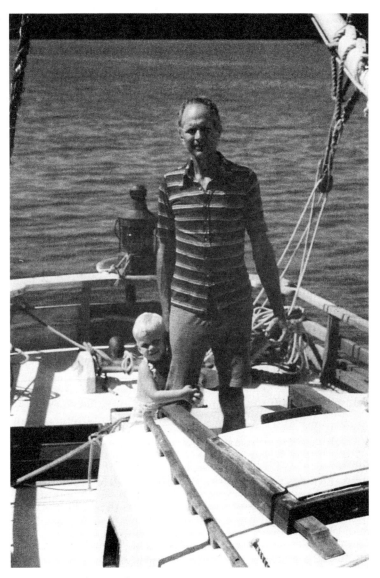

*Peter and Thomas Tangvald onboard L'Artemis, taken by the police in a
reconstruction of the view that the pirates had of Thomas clinging to Peter's leg*

Brunei, which they reached on 27 February, where Peter's troubles really began.

Thomas was taken to hospital and Peter began an interminable series of police interrogations, each time with a different team. These were spread over two weeks. It was clear the police were suspicious of Peter's story and one day when ashore he was appalled to see a newspaper headline saying: 'Pirate Attack or the (Nearly) Perfect Matrimonial Murder?' The police next questioned Thomas without Peter being present. A police photographer came on board *L'Artemis* where they recorded a reconstruction of the incident with a model standing in for Lydia. Eventually Peter was told that his case was closed and he was free to leave. A friendly policeman told Peter the problem was that the police had been suspicious as to why he had not been shot too and the boat sunk. He said there were some 300 pirate attacks each year and that normally the pirates shot everyone on board, took everything from the boat which they then sank with the bodies locked inside.

Peter's first reaction after his release was to try to sell the *L'Artemis* and go home to Europe or the USA with Thomas. But he could not find a buyer. Then he tried to find a crew to help him sail the boat back to Europe but no-one suitable came forward.

Left with no alternative and determined to get to sea again, Peter left Brunei in April with only Thomas on board. They headed for the Malacca Strait and the Indian Ocean. They passed Singapore at night and on 2 May dropped anchor outside Malacca's breakwater. The next day they moved into the harbour.

At that time of year, the monsoon was blowing the wrong

way across the Indian Ocean and Peter knew he would have to wait for eight or nine months for the north easterly monsoon to return. Peter managed to enrol Thomas in a Salvation Army school where Peter met the Chinese headmistress. Peter liked Malaya and its people and began to regain his strength and some of his equilibrium.

One morning Peter got a surprise and received perhaps the best medicine possible. He heard a distinguished British voice hailing him from the quay, "Ahoy, *L'Artemis*, ahoy." It was his old friend Edward Allcard, now in his 60s and with a snow white beard. He had flown from the Seychelles to see what he could do to help. As soon as Edward heard the news of what had happened to his old friend, he had boarded an aeroplane to Malaya, leaving his wife Clare to watch their ship. He stayed a few days and they talked about old times and the future. Edward's visit helped Peter's recovery and made his outlook on life much brighter.

Tangvald worked out that the best time to leave for the west would be in late December when the winds would be favourable. Early that month he went to the school to tell the headmistress, who he had got to know a little, that he would be taking Thomas away and they would be leaving the island. She said to Peter that it would be much better if he took a woman with him. Peter agreed but said he knew of no-one who would go with him. She replied, "You're wrong. You know at least one such woman – me." Peter stood completely dumbfounded whilst she went on to say that she would make a good wife to him and please would he wait thirty days before leaving so she could work out her notice at the school. Peter learnt she was called Ann Ho San Chew and was 32 years old.

On 2 January 1980 Ann came on board with all her posses-
sions and remained with Peter for many years. They set sail that
day for Sri Lanka arriving at the end of January. There they
met three tourists who asked to join the ship as paying crew.
Reluctantly Peter took them on, persuaded by Ann who said
they could do with the money. They left on 10 February to cross
the Indian Ocean. The crew were little help, disregarded orders,
complained about Ann's cooking and the safety of the ship. Peter
decided to get rid of them as soon as possible and land them at
the first suitable port they came to. This was to be Djibouti, now
independent from France.

L'Artemis arrived on 4 March and Peter disembarked the three
crew members without bothering with any formalities or obtaining clearance to enter or leave the country. Peter did not appreciate that Djibouti was no longer a relaxed French outpost
but was now a new fiercely independent country with a totally
different attitude to incomers. *L'Artemis* left the main harbour
and found a secluded lagoon in the outer part of the anchorage
where they stayed for four days, completely hidden from view
among the mangroves. Later Peter and Ann learnt of their very
narrow escape. The paying crew had gone to Immigration and
Customs and told them they had been put ashore by a foreign
yacht which had then left without any clearance. Straight away
the Immigration people set out to catch and arrest Peter and
Ann for the crime of smuggling aliens into their country. A warship was sent to intercept them but found no trace of the yacht
anywhere out at sea. They were, of course, lying hidden just in
front of the town where no-one bothered to look. Had *L'Artemis*
been found, Peter and Ann would have been thrown into gaol
and the yacht impounded and probably lost for ever.

They had a hard trip up the Red Sea. Not only did the prevailing northerly headwinds blow strongly most of the time, but they were troubled by Egyptian soldiers everywhere they stopped. *L'Artemis* was rammed and badly damaged by the Egyptian customs launch at Suez and once again Peter had to take an expensive tow through the canal.

With much relief at getting away from Egypt they headed into the Mediterranean. They reached Larnaca in Cyprus three days later and spent the summer in and amongst the Greek islands. In the autumn they sailed to Tunisia planning to spend the winter there. They found it hard to find a sheltered harbour with protection from the winter gales but in November they moored in the small fishing harbour of Gabes. One night, soon after their arrival, Peter and Ann, asleep in their bunk, were awoken by three knife-yielding intruders who demanded money. Peter was tied up and badly beaten. They then attempted to rape Ann but, screaming and fighting, she successfully fought them off. The attackers fled with all of their money and all of Ann's jewellery. The police found the attackers but none of their stolen belongings were ever returned. To make matters worse they were told their three-month visa would not be extended; this would normally have been a mere formality. The judge appointed for the trial of the attackers was most unhelpful and would not assist Peter in any way, refusing to interfere in the matter of the visa. They therefore had to leave the port before the trial and well before the end of the winter storms. Peter was convinced that, in exchange for their freedom, the criminals had surrendered the jewellery and money, which was then split between the police and the judge.

On 21 March 1981 they left Tunisia and headed towards

Europe. Their first port of call was Cagliari in Sardinia where they lingered amongst friends for nearly four months. After the attack in Tunisia, Peter and Ann had agreed they really should sell the boat and settle down, buying a house somewhere they liked. They decided to try Norway, where Peter had family, and in July they put back to sea intending to sail there.

They stopped in Portugal and then sailed non-stop to Falmouth. Rather than try to get to Norway just before the cold weather set in, they spent the winter afloat in the Helford River, just south of Falmouth. In the spring Peter was lent a car in which they drove to Norway where, in May, he and Ann got married. In Norway, Ann had never been so cold in all her life and, after looking at the country through tropical eyes, the couple decided that it, and a life away from the sea, was not for them. They headed back to England.

Back in Cornwall, they prepared *L'Artemis* for a transatlantic trip and left on 25 July for the Canary Islands. Averaging 140 miles per day they arrived on 4 August. They left in September and headed for French Guiana which they reached on 10 October. The country had changed considerably since Peter was last there. Excessive French bureaucracy frightened off Peter from setting up a boatyard, which had been at the back of his mind for many years. Ann was not happy there as too many of the people she met remembered Simonne and Lydia. Despite this they lingered for a while and enrolled Thomas in a local school.

Just before Christmas they sailed to Martinique, where Ann announced that she was pregnant. They moved on to Antigua, where Peter tried to get a residents permit for Ann to enter the United States. This proved impossible. Giving up the idea of

America they headed back to Europe, arriving in the Azores on 15 July 1983. Onward they went to Spain and then Portugal ending up in Faro, where Ann gave birth (in a proper hospital this time) to their daughter. They named her Carmen.

They stayed in Faro for the winter in a safe berth above a railway bridge which had to be dismantled to let the yacht through. The family spent virtually the whole of the next year amongst the harbours of Portugal and Spain until the onset of cold autumn winds reminded them that winter was approaching. In November *L'Artemis* set sail back toward the Caribbean, stopping only at the Canary Islands on the way.

On 26 January 1985 they were nearing Grenada in the West Indies when tragedy struck *L'Artemis* once again. Ann, whilst on deck hanging up some washing, was caught unawares when the boat suddenly gybed. Peter shouted a warning to Ann but it was too late and the heavy main boom swung across hitting her and flinging her far overboard. No trace of her was ever found despite a long search. After six hours Thomas spotted something in the water but it was only the bucket Ann had been using for her washing. They gave up the search and sailed on.

On 29 January Peter anchored in St George's Harbour in Grenada, desperately sad and alone with just two small children. Thomas was seven and Carmen just over a year old.

In despair, Peter decided to sail *L'Artemis* to Annapolis in the USA where he would sell her and settle ashore. With only Thomas to help him, they set off first for Beaufort in North Carolina and then northward through the intra-coastal waterway. A week later, as they neared Norfolk in Virginia, fate intervened which stopped them in their tracks. They went no further north.

That day a Belgian yacht, with only a father and daughter on board, moored alongside *L'Artemis*. Peter and Thomas were invited on board for dinner. After the meal, the daughter Florence, who said she was 18 years old, announced that she would rather sail with Peter on a boat with no engine than continue with her father. He raised no objection almost encouraging her; he was probably much happier to carry on alone. Florence jumped ship and turned out to be a good crew, cook and nanny for the children.

All thoughts of selling *L'Artemis* soon disappeared, so they turned around and headed south. On 21 September 1985 they arrived in San Juan on Puerto Rico, just in time to avoid hurricane Gloria. Four days later Florence and Peter were married. Florence was Peter's seventh (and last) wife. In October the next year Florence gave birth to a daughter, Virginia. She was born on board *L'Artemis* on the same settee where Thomas had been born.

Three years later Florence's parents wanted her back home and persuaded her to leave Peter and go back to Canada with her daughter. When told this, Peter became so distraught that he had a near fatal heart attack and was in hospital in intensive care for twelve days. He never saw Florence or his daughter Virginia again.

Believing that he did not have long to live, Peter wrote to his old friend Edward Allcard saying how worried he was about the future for Thomas and Carmen if he should die. Clare Allcard told Edward to write back saying that Peter was not to worry and, if anything should happen, they, the Allcards, would take care of the children. Peter then made a will appointing Edward and Clare to be the children's guardians.

For the next three years *L'Artemis* stayed in Puerto Rico and Thomas and Carmen attended a local school. Thomas, who had spent his whole life on board *L'Artemis* and knew nothing else, now acquired his own boat, a 22-foot gaff sloop designed by the American Howard Chapelle, with the very appropriate name of *Spartan*.

By 1991 Peter was 67 years old and not in good health. But he became restless once more and wanted to move on. He decided to sail for Bonaire, an island in the Dutch Antilles. Many people tried to stop him going with just his two children and without any other crew to help. When Edward Allcard heard what Tangvald was proposing, he wrote to Peter pleading with him not to set off with only seven-year-old Carmen on board. His timing was also considered very unwise as he was planning to leave in the middle of the hurricane season. Despite this they set off on 18 July 1991 with Peter and Carmen on *L'Artemis* and Thomas on *Spartan* at the end of a 300-foot nylon tow rope. The passage was uneventful until they approached Bonaire in the early hours of 22 July when Peter inexplicably ran *L'Artemis* onto a coral reef some 30 miles to windward of their destination.

The epilogue to Peter's autobiography, *At Any Cost*, which was published posthumously, contains the following description of what happened next, written by his son Thomas:

I suddenly saw three rocks jutting out of the horizon and thought 'Oh, no! This must be Aves' (a dangerous coral atoll some 30 miles to windward of Bonaire). Then I saw the broad white line, the boiling foam of relentless, charging waves crashing onto the shore.

In seconds L'Artemis was on it, the bow plunging down and the stern rising with such violence as to knock all the wind out of the main. "Non! Non!" I screamed, as if it were going to make any difference. It can't be real, I thought, it must be a particularly large wave. But when I noticed the limp towline, I knew this was the real thing. I looked at my Dad's 50-foot boat being tossed about like a piece of driftwood in the surf. The boat set itself parallel to the coast. The next instant the rig snapped off with a crack audible above the thunder of the roaring waves.

I rushed inside, fumbling with the knot, frantically trying to untie my surfboard in complete darkness, for there was no moon at all. Once free, I shoved it in the cockpit and groped for a pair of pants, found none and gave up, leaving only in a wool shirt and rain jacket. I jumped in the water with my surfboard, paddling for Dad's boat, wanting to be with them and to scramble ashore together. But when I got closer, I was afraid of getting crushed by the boat.

I stayed as close to L'Artemis as possible, waiting for a break in the waves to dash in and jump ashore. Under the light of the stern lamp, I could see the boat being destroyed with ghastly efficiency. She would leap in the air with the rising water and, as the water went back out, the boat would drop 10 feet onto the sharp coral with the sickening noise of cracking wood and my sister's hysterical screams coming from inside. For a minute or two, I saw my Dad sitting in the companionway shining a flashlight out to sea and then across the reef. I put my surfboard up in the air, but I don't think he saw me.

Then L'Artemis's stern lamp went out from the successive shocks, leaving her completely in the dark. I paddled out and away from the breaking waves. After a little while, I didn't feel panic at all. Instead it was a lot like a dream. I figured I just had to keep paddling to stay warm, and wait until sunrise when I could climb the coral and find them both waiting for me.

After some three hours, the sun finally came up and I could see the coast. At around 9 o'clock, I finally got on shore without too many scratches but, after staying six hours on the surfboard, I had massive friction burns. Immediately I set out searching for my father and sister – but they weren't there.

Peter's body was recovered straight away but Carmen's was not found until much later. It will never be known why Peter ran onto the reef but it could well be that he had a heart or angina attack, which incapacitated him. An empty ampoule of nitro-glycerine, used to ease the pain of such attacks, was found in the wreckage.

*

Thomas was 15 years old and arrived on the island of Bonaire traumatised and quite alone in the world. He had seen his mother shot, his step mother knocked overboard and lost and now his father and half-sister had drowned. He was taken in by a priest whom he told about the man with the white beard who had come to visit them in Malaya some years before. The priest tracked down the Allcards to their eyrie in Andorra, who straight away flew out to Bonaire and took Thomas back home with them. Edward was then 75 years old and Clare, his wife, was 45. They had only recently settled in Andorra after a lifetime of wandering the world's oceans, all wonderfully recorded in their various books about their travels and life at sea.

Recently I visited the Allcards in their home high in the

Pyrenean mountains. Edward is now 102 and still fit and in remarkable health. He only gave up skiing at 96 when someone
skied into him and shattered one of his knees. Clare, a well-
known author, is now 70. They told me Thomas's story.

*

Thomas was extremely bright and had already been found
to have an IQ of 148. On arrival in Andorra, Clare enrolled
Thomas in a local Lycée. He spent three years there before winning a British Gas scholarship to Leeds University. He refused a
place at Cambridge University because he said he could not study
in a college where signs declared 'KEEP OFF THE GRASS'.
He graduated from Leeds with a degree in Mathematics and
Fluid Dynamics. Whilst at Leeds he bought, with some of his
British Gas scholarship money, an old 22-foot wooden Itchen
Ferry called *Melody*. Thomas followed in his father's footsteps by
buying a boat which was gaff-rigged, had no engine and was
extremely simple and spartan.

After working for a while in Cornwall, Thomas sailed *Melody*
single-handed and non-stop to Culebra in Puerto Rico. There
he met an American girl called Christina and they soon married.
After their son Gaston was born they settled on a small farm on
Vieques, a small island off Puerto Rico's north-eastern coast.

Thomas next bought a traditional 34-foot open cockpit
Puerto Rican engine-less fishing smack called *Oasis*. Thomas
and his father had seen and admired the boat some years before when Thomas had declared he would one day own her. He
made many modifications to make the boat fit for ocean sailing. These included building a cabin over the front of the cock-

pit, cutting down the sail plan and converting her to gaff rig. In 2012 Thomas, with a heavily pregnant Christina and their son Gaston, set sail in *Oasis* for Brazil where they wanted Christina to give birth. If they did this, their new child would have Brazilian nationality which would permit Thomas to buy some land there. They achieved their aim and Lucio was born soon after arrival.

Thomas could not find any work in Brazil so they moved on to French Guiana where work of a sort was available. In 2013 Christina and the children went back to the Caribbean where Christina tried to get US citizenship for Lucio but without success. She was told to apply through the US Embassy back in the country where Lucio had been born.

Meanwhile Thomas continued working at Cayenne in French Guiana designing and helping to build fishing boats. He hauled *Oasis* ashore for a refit. He removed all the ballast and stored it alongside her. It was all promptly stolen. Thomas had no money to replace it but gradually collected some old pieces of iron to use instead. But he never collected enough and *Oasis* was relaunched woefully under ballasted.

Thomas came up with a plan for him and his family to settle on the Ile de Noronho off the coast of Brazil where he would pursue his work as a naval architect. He decided to sail there in *Oasis* to find out what it was like and whether his plan was feasible. On 4 March 2014 he set off alone in *Oasis* on a 1,500-mile passage to the island.

Thomas and *Oasis* never arrived and no sign of them has ever been found. He was 37 years old.

Chapter 10

The Life and Last Voyage of Eric Tabarly on board his Yacht *Pen Duick* (1998)

The name 'Eric Tabarly'. Where to start? Sailor, French naval officer, innovator, creative genius, father figure, role model, rule bender (rule cheat to some), fierce competitor, inspiration to a whole generation, scourge of the yachting establishment, family man, author and lots more besides.

The name '*Pen Duick*', forever associated with Tabarly. Where to start? A bird – the word means 'swallow' in Breton. Six yachts, each one more innovative than the one before. The first, bought by Eric's father in 1938, when Eric was seven, decommissioned during World War II for fear of her being requisitioned, rebuilt after the war, kept and treasured ever after by the Tabarly family. Five more followed bearing the name *Pen Duick*, all inspired by Eric, all made history and all were winners of most of the major sailing trophies around the world.

Eric Tabarly was single-handedly responsible for the present unchallenged predominance of France in the world of long distance ocean racing. Today, large and expensive sailing machines of one, two or three hulls, some flying over the waves on foils, charge around the world's ocean race courses bearing such names as Banque Populaire, Groupama, Credit Agricole, Castorama, Sodebo and those of other large prestigious French companies. Each year these companies pour millions of euros into campaigning these boats. Their skippers have become household names, treated (and paid) like rock stars. Before Tabarly came along, the British ruled these particular waves and did so in a much more understated way.

The speed of these new creations is truly amazing. The ultimate ocean race of them all, the single-handed non-stop round the world Vendée Globe Race is run every four years. From France to France around the world's three southerly capes (the Cape of Good Hope, Cape Leeuwin and Cape Horn), the race has seen overall times reduce from 109 days in 1989 to 78 days in 2012. Imagine sailing a fast uncomfortable 60-foot carbon fibre skimming dish, not unlike an overgrown dinghy, right round the world, down the Atlantic Ocean, across the Equator into the Southern Ocean, through the Roaring Forties, then around the feared Cape Horn and back up the Atlantic to France: all without stopping. And alone. Eighty days and nights without a break through some of the most dangerous waters in the world. To do this you have to keep up an average speed of around 20 knots or around 24 miles per hour, twenty-four hours a day, seven days a week.

But these are just the monohulls. The speeds reached by the latest generation of monster French multihulls are truly staggering. The largest trimaran currently sailing, *Spindrift 2*, previously known as *Banque Populaire*, is 120 feet long and regularly reaches speeds of 50 knots or more, has crossed the Atlantic in under 6 days (about the time the largest ocean liners used to take) and has sailed around the world in 45 days. These speeds would have been unthinkable a few years ago when the Jules Verne Trophy was first proposed for any boat that could sail around the world in under 80 days. It took many attempts before anyone did it and now the time taken has been nearly halved. Using technology developed for the latest America's Cup catamarans, the French have begun to fit foils to their ocean going trimarans which can now 'fly' at 30 knots upwind and well over 50 knots downwind, that is nearly 58 miles per hour. Without Tabarly, none of this might have happened.

Eric Tabarly was born in Brittany in 1931. His parents were Bretons and Eric was educated in and lived his entire life in Brittany. He was born in Nantes on 24 July 1931 to a family with the sea in their blood. As a baby his parents took him sailing on their 9 metre cutter *Annie* and in 1938, when Eric was seven, his father bought a yacht which was old even then. She was called *Pen Duick* and had been designed and built in 1898 in Scotland by the legendary yacht designer William Fife at his yard in Fairlie on the River Clyde. She was 48 feet long, rigged as a gaff cutter with the then fashionable schooner bow. Like all of Fife's boats, she was elegant, seaworthy and fast. Despite being in an appalling state, Eric's father was seduced by the boat's beauty and bought her.

Eric liked sailing from the start but, above all, loved sailing on *Pen Duick*, which remained with him all his life. He did not like school or shine there. He disappointed his parents who dreamed of Eric joining the French Navy and becoming an Admiral.

A year after the Tabarlys had bought *Pen Duick*, the Second World War broke out. Eric's father was called up and the boat was laid up. After his father departed for the war, Eric's mother moved Eric, his two sisters and younger brother to her parents' house in the village of Prefailles, near the mouth of the river Loire on the western coast of France. Despite the privations of the war and the German occupation, Eric enjoyed his time there, save for the food shortages and his schooling, which did not go well.

At the end of the war, when his father was demobilised, he and Eric went to see how *Pen Duick* had survived. Not at all well was the answer. Eric was minded of a melancholy old dog, sick and abandoned. But she was in one piece and nobody had taken off the iron ballast keel, which had happened to many boats in France. They set out to refit the old yacht and began to cruise her again during the summer months. They based her in the yachting harbour of La Trinité-sur-Mer. There they put the boat in the hands of the Costantini family who ran a shipyard and who later played an important part in the Tabarly story.

In 1947 Eric's father, Guy, who was a textile fabric salesman, was in financial difficulties and he laid up the boat once more. In 1952 he told the family he could no longer afford to keep *Pen Duick* and she would have to be sold. Eric, who was then 21 years old, was shocked and, as he was starting in the Navy the next year, he told his father that he would scrape by and save his wages for as long as needed if they could keep the boat. His father agreed and passed the boat on to Eric. So Tabarly became the owner of his first boat.

On joining the Navy, Eric was assigned to the Fleet Air Arm and learnt to fly. He did not enjoy his training but eventually passed out as a qualified pilot. He served as a pilot in French airbases in Morocco and in 1954 flew in the First French-Indochina War.

In 1956 he returned to France and went back to La Trinité-sur-Mer to talk to Gilles Costantini about refitting *Pen Duick*. Gilles told Eric that the boat was rotten, had had it and couldn't be repaired. After much thought Eric decided to use the hull of *Pen Duick* as a mould, round which he would build a new hull out of fibreglass. Eric set to, doing most of the work himself over weekends and during his leave periods. It took two years. In the autumn of 1958 the new hull was floated out of the boatyard and turned the right way up, the old wooden hull on the inside was demolished and taken out and a new deck was fitted. Eric did not have the money to pay for all of this but Gilles told Eric he could sort that out when he was able. "Pay us when you can", they said to Eric many times.

The next year Eric got his longed for place at the French Naval College in Brest and he started on a two-year course. He spent whatever time he could preparing and then sailing his beloved *Pen Duick*. On his first voyage, the mast broke and damaged the boat; Tabarly did not have the money to buy a new one. A few days later Gilles telephoned Eric to say a benefactor, who wanted to remain anonymous, had agreed to pay for all the repairs. Eric was sure he knew who this was but never disclosed the person's identity.

During his two years at the Naval College, Eric was given much time off to sail and, with the Commandant's approval, took many of his fellow cadets out with him. The Commandant appreciated that not only was this good training for the cadets but that sailing was really the only thing Tabarly was any good for.

At the conclusion of his course Eric went on a tour of the world on the French training vessel *Jeanne d'Arc* and, on their return to Brest, Eric saw close to them a yacht under full sail – it was *Pen Duick*, with his father at the helm and his brother, Patrick, at his side. *Jeanne d'Arc* raised her tricolour as a salute.

Following his commission, Eric was posted to Cherbourg. He moved *Pen Duick* to Normandy, assembled a strong crew, which included his father and his brother, who was 13 years younger than him, and looked for some races to enter. There was virtually no ocean racing taking place in France at that time, so Eric looked across the Channel to France's old adversary, Great Britain, where such racing had become well established. This had all started with the first Fastnet Race in 1925, won coincidentally by a French-built but English-owned yacht, *Jolie Brise*. England had made this sport her own and the French were nowhere to be seen.

Eric took *Pen Duick* across the Channel and, in 1960, took part in the Channel Race, the Cowes-La Coruna Race, the Irish Sea Race and the Fastnet Race (from which they had to retire with torn sails).

In June 1962 Eric read about a British organised single-handed Transatlantic race, which had become known as the OSTAR, the second running of which was to start from Plymouth on 23 May 1964. The first race had been held in 1960 with five entrants and had been won by Francis Chichester in this boat *Gipsy Moth III*. Tabarly became determined to enter the 1964 race and win it. He just needed to decide on what boat to take. The old *Pen Duick*, with her heavy gaff rig, was not suitable and Eric headed to Brittany to talk to his old friend Gilles Costantini about the possibility of building a new yacht designed specifically for the race.

Gilles and his brother agreed to build one at their own expense, which they would lend to Eric for the race. Work began in October 1962 on a light displacement 10 metre yacht to be called *Margilic V*. She was launched in April 1963 and Eric took her on several offshore races. Eric soon realised that he could easily manage a much larger (and thereby faster) boat and persuaded the Costantinis that what he really needed for the OSTAR was a bigger and stronger one. After much discussion, plans were drawn up for a longer version. She was to be built out of plywood with a multi-chined hull and a long counter. She was to be ketch rigged to keep all sails a manageable size. Tabarly did not have any money to pay for such a boat but the Costantinis again came to his rescue. They agreed to sell *Margilic V* and put the proceeds toward the cost of this new one. Eric was to find the rest of the money, when he could.

Work started in January 1964, only five months before the start of the race. The boat was 13.60 metres long (44 feet), with a draught of 2.20 metres and a beam of 3.40 metres. She was launched on 5 April and the bare hull taken to the French Naval shipyard at Lorient, where the French Navy had agreed to finish her off. The work was completed and she was officially named on 9 May 1964 as *Pen Duick II*. There was barely time to rig and fit the sails and mount the self- steering gear before Tabarly had to leave for Plymouth, which he did on 16 May.

Tabarly arrived at Millbay Dock in Plymouth two days later and immediately began to assess his rivals. The first he observed was Francis Chichester, who was sailing the race again in his faithful *Gipsy Moth III*. Most of the other entries were heavy conventional cruising boats, seaworthy and slow but able to cope with heavy weather. There was a smattering of multihulls and, of course, Blondie Hasler, the originator of the race, in his junk rigged Folkboat *Jester*.

The other competitors were intrigued by *Pen Duick II*, many wondering whether she was too light, too fragile and too big for one man to handle. Tabarly for his part was determined to beat Britain at her own game.

Before the start it soon became clear that the race was really to be a needle match between Chichester and Tabarly, between England and France. Chichester, attired as ever in double breasted navy blazer and club tie, was a picture of calm and good organisation against the young quietly-spoken Breton naval officer frantically trying to get his steed ready as the last pieces of equipment were fitted and made to work.

After a poor start Tabarly soon overtook Chichester and led a procession down the English Channel to the open Atlantic. The weather threw up the usual brew of westerly gales, followed by periods of light winds with fog but, along with these, there was a fair share of favourable easterly winds. Tabarly experienced a series of problems but kept the boat sailing fast. First his self-steering gear gave up but he soon learnt how to trim the sails to keep *Pen Duick II* on course. He spent long hours at the helm, getting little sleep. Then his halyards at the masthead came adrift requiring him to climb the mast, a perilous thing to do when alone on a boat pitching and rolling in an Atlantic swell.

Tabarly arrived at the finish line by the Nantucket lightship at 10.45 on the morning of 18 June, in a time of 27 days and 4 hours. Chichester arrived two days later, having taken 29 days, compared to the 40 days he took in the first race. On his arrival Chichester gave Tabarly a warm handshake and said, "It is an honour to have been beaten by a sailor such as you."

The whole of France went wild for Tabarly. Not only had a Frenchman beaten the English, but they now had a new hero in this 32-year-old naval officer. 'A Breton now rules the waves', as one newspaper put it. In entering this race Tabarly had only two

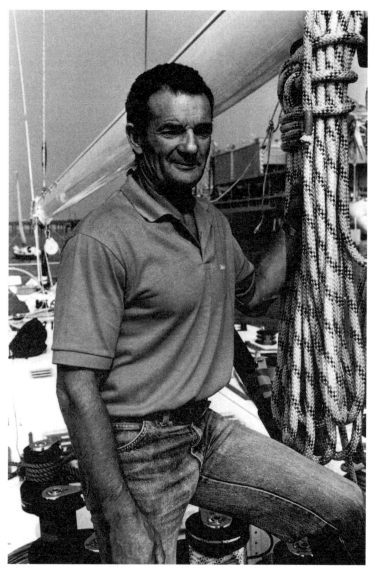

Eric Tabarly on board Cote D'Or at the start of the
1985 Whitbread Round the World Race

ambitions – to cross the Atlantic single-handed and to beat the English. He had achieved both.

After the race Tabarly was taken to Washington where the French Ambassador presented him with the Legion d'Honneur, France's top award. Eric then sailed *Pen Duick II* to New York where the boat was loaded onto a cargo ship for a free trip back to France. Tabarly was given free passage home on the liner *France*.

Tabarly then went back to normal naval duties until late in 1965, when he was seconded to the Department of the Minister for Sports and Young People. The Minister was the famous French mountaineering hero Maurice Herzog, the first man to climb Annapurna in the Himalayas, the first 8,000 metre mountain to be climbed. This position allowed Tabarly almost total freedom to pursue his sailing ambitions whilst receiving a naval officer's pay. The Department agreed to buy *Pen Duick II* for its sailing school in Brittany on the basis that Tabarly could continue to use her whenever he wanted.

Next, Tabarly put together a close group of young French disciples to crew for him. They followed him from race to race and from boat to boat. Many of these young men went on to become successful and famous skippers themselves. They formed a nucleus of a group of French sailors who developed this new sport of sailing. They became as well-known as rock stars and, in years to come, attracted millions of euros in sponsorship money to build a succession of ever faster and more extreme boats to race across the world's oceans. New races to far flung destinations were established, often with heavy sponsorship money, leading inevitably to the ultimate – a single handed non-stop race around the world. France is now at the very pinnacle of this sport and many thousands of people all over France have been attracted by those people's antics to take up sailing.

Two years after the OSTAR, Tabarly took *Pen Duick II* once again across the Atlantic to participate in the bi-annual Newport to Bermuda race, then he raced her back across the Atlantic to Copenhagen. Back in France, Eric was once more out of money but started to plan for *Pen Duick III*, a much larger yacht to be built out of aluminium. Somehow the money was found and the boat was launched in May 1967. This boat caused controversy with its unusual schooner rig, taking advantage of some loopholes which Tabarly discovered in the English rating rules. In England this was considered unsportsmanlike and the yacht was thought of as a travesty. *Pen Duick III* was selected as one of the French three-boat team for the British-run Admiral's Cup, then considered the Grand Prix of ocean racing. *Pen Duick III* won all three races, including the Fastnet race. Later in the season *Pen Duick III* also won the Plymouth-La Rochelle race and the La Rochelle to Benodet race. After that the boat was shipped to Australia to take part in the annual Sydney to Hobart Race, in which she won her class. Tabarly, his crew and boat returned to France in triumph. Nobody, especially in France, had seen results like this before.

Back in England, and as a result of these successes, the Royal Ocean Racing Club, who then made the rating rules, promptly changed them to plug these loopholes. No longer would a schooner have any chance of winning anything. Tabarly was very unhappy about this and made his displeasure well known. He had to re-rig his boat as a ketch for the next year's season.

Before they returned to Europe they took *Pen Duick III* on a cruise to New Caledonia. A young French language teacher at Sydney University asked if he could come along with them. Tabarly asked the man his name; he replied, "Alain Colas." He joined them and remained with Tabarly for many years. As we saw in Chapter 5, Colas went on to become famous (and infamous) in his own right.

Tabarly now began to consider the 1968 OSTAR and came to believe that the race could only be won by a multihull. He therefore commissioned the building of a revolutionary trimaran to be built out of aluminium. Again, lack of money held up construction but Tabarly was just able to raise sufficient funds from selling his story to a number of French TV and magazine companies.

The new boat, to become *Pen Duick IV*, was 67 feet long, with a beam of 35 feet. The three hulls were held together by a series of aluminium struts and the whole had the appearance of some strange piece of agricultural machinery. In France she soon became known as 'the floating tennis court' and in England was referred to as 'the sea spider'. She was designed by Frenchman Andre Allegre who was in the forefront of multihull development at that time. She was ketch rigged and was one of the first multihulls to have rotating wing masts and a fully battened mainsail and mizzen. Due to delays in the construction she was not launched until 11 May, only some 10 days before the start of the race. Inevitably with such a radical design Tabarly suffered many teething troubles and the boat was in no fit state to start the race. Tabarly did not get far. On the first night at sea he narrowly avoided a collision then, at three o'clock in the morning, he went below to have some coffee. He had not been below for more than fifteen minutes when he collided with a cargo vessel. The starboard float was damaged and the forward compartment holed. Tabarly considered carrying on until midday the next day, when a mizzen shroud broke. With the mast likely to come tumbling down at any moment, Tabarly turned and headed back to Plymouth.

He had the damage repaired and four days later set off again. He was no luckier this time. Very soon the self-steering gear broke down and Tabarly could barely turn the rudder. He put into nearby Newlyn on the Cornish coast, repaired the damage and set off the next day. A few miles out it all broke again. This time Tabarly was finished with the race and he turned the boat home toward France.

That same year Tabarly heard about a proposed single-handed Transpacific race, being organised by the American Slocum Society. The race was to start on 15 March 1969 and the course was to be from San Francisco Bay to the entrance of the bay of Tokyo, a distance of some 5,000 miles. Surprisingly, the race was for monohulls only with a maximum length of 35 feet. Tabarly was tempted to enter. He studied the route and the likely winds to be experienced and decided that he needed a completely new kind of vessel capable of prolonged fast downwind sailing. In conjunction with naval architect Michel Bigoin, they came up with the idea of a lightweight very wide skimming dish to be held upright partly by a small ballast keel but principally by water ballast which could be pumped into and out of large tanks along the sides of the boat. This was a new innovation which has now been universally adopted in today's long distance short-handed races. The final design was for a yacht 35 feet long with a beam of 11 feet – a huge amount for boats of that day – a draft of 7 feet 6 inches with a displacement varying between 3.2 and 3.7 tons, depending on the amount of water ballast taken on board.

She was built out of aluminium and proved to be a very light boat capable of planing at high speeds, just like a racing dinghy.

Building started in October 1968 and the boat, named *Pen Duick V*, was launched in November. She was put onto a cargo ship to be delivered to San Francisco in time to start the race in March the next year.

Never liking to be idle, Tabarly used this interlude to sail his trimaran *Pen Duick IV* across the Atlantic to try her out properly and maybe find a buyer in the USA. The wing masts were abandoned and new standard masts were fitted. The self-steering gear was sorted out. On 26 November 1968 Tabarly, with Olivier de Kersauson and Alain Colas as crew, left La Trinité-sur-Mer and arrived in Martinique on 19 December, having called in at Tenerife. They made a record Atlantic crossing in ten and a half days. They then traversed the Panama Canal on 2 February 1969 and set sail for San Francisco.

In March 1969 *Pen Duick V* was unloaded from the cargo ship, five days before the start of the race, leaving Tabarly no real time to prepare the boat properly. There were five competitors in the race, one of whom was fellow Frenchman Jean Yves Terlain. He became famous later in the annals of the OSTAR.

Conditions were good at the start and Tabarly was leading the fleet by the time they passed under the Golden Gate Bridge. He decided to take a south westerly route to pass close to Hawaii and then to swing north west to Japan. This route was not the shortest but it gave the best chances of favourable winds. Tabarly was proved right and he had good conditions with only the odd period of bad weather. All went well on board with a minimum of problems or breakages and he often found himself surfing over the waves in a spectacular manner.

On 24 April Tabarly was the first to cross the finish line, having taken 39 days and 15 hours. Jean Yves Terlain arrived second after a further ten days, a good performance in a much slower boat.

Leaving his skimming dish in Tokyo to be shipped back to France, Tabarly joined his crew on *Pen Duick IV* and they took part in the Los Angeles-Honolulu race where they comfortably outstripped all opposition including the mighty *Windward Passage*, a formidable racing machine and, at that time, one of the fastest yachts in the world. Tabarly then continued with *Pen Duick IV* across the Pacific looking for a buyer. None could be found until they were in Nouméa when, as described in Chapter 5, crew member Alain Colas announced he had fallen in love with the trimaran and wanted to buy her. After Colas had scrabbled around for the money she became his, with Tabarly's blessing.

Next came the first Whitbread fully crewed Round the World Race due to start in September 1973. Tabarly wanted to build a new boat but serious money was required which proved difficult to come by. He began to realise he was going to have to start taking his fund raising more seriously in the future. He therefore appointed an agent in Paris who came up with the necessary funds just in time. The French naval architect Andre Mauric was commissioned to design a new yacht capable of winning the race. Plans were only finalised in November 1972, less than a year before the start and Tabarly struggled to find a yard able to build the boat in the time available. Eventually, and as was becoming the norm, the French Navy stepped in and agreed to build it at the Naval shipyard in Brest.

At the end of July 1973 the new vessel, *Pen Duick VI*, was ready for sea trials. Tabarly's first race was the Fastnet race in which,

despite a very poor and late start, they finished in ninth position, way ahead of all their future Whitbread Round the World
competitors. It was then that rumours began to spread that the
French Navy had used depleted uranium from their nuclear sub-
marines for the ballast keel, instead of the usual lead. Some people thought that, as this material was heavier than lead, it would
give *Pen Duick VI* a big advantage over her competitors. In fact,
the reason for its use was that Tabarly had run out of money
and he was given this material for free by the French Navy. Less
uranium was needed than the equivalent weight of lead so there
was no weight advantage.

When the Whitbread fleet assembled for the start line off
Portsmouth, Tabarly for once felt at ease and well prepared. He
had assembled a strong twelve-man crew. By nightfall on the first
day of the race, only Chay Blyth's *Great Britain II* (on which boat
Rob James was sailing) remained in sight. On 4 October when
everything pointed to *Pen Duick VI* being likely to be first to Cape
Town, the first stop of the race, the mast came down – broken
at the lower spreaders. The crew cut away the broken bits, used
the boom as a jury mast and, under a much reduced rig, set sail
for Rio de Janeiro. Tabarly contacted his shore team by radio
who persuaded the French Ministry of Defence to fly a new mast
out to Rio. A plane was made available which could take off the
next day.

Pen Duick VI arrived in Rio ten days after the dismasting. The
crew stepped the new mast, set up the rigging and strengthened
the deck underneath it. Tabarly believed a weakness there may
have led to the breakage. They left Rio on 20 October with 3,250
miles to go to get to Cape Town in time to re-join the race. After
15 days and 19 hours they crossed the finishing line to be told

that they had just smashed the Rio-Cape Town record.

The next leg of the race to Sydney restarted on 7 November, only a few hours after Tabarly and his crew had arrived. *Pen Duick VI* soon took the lead and they sailed the boat hard across the Indian Ocean, the only damage being some blown out sails. They arrived first in Sydney.

On 29 December they started on the third leg to Rio de Janeiro. The next day disaster struck again. The new mast, mainsail and boom came crashing onto the deck. The race was over for them and they motored back to Sydney. A third mast was fitted and the boat was sailed back home to France. The next year, 1974, the mast broke yet again.

In 1975 Tabarly put together a new crew including the then unknowns Eric Loiseau, Phillipe Poupon and Titouan Lamazou, all of whom would later carve out names for themselves as skippers of their own boats. They joined Tabarly for the 1975 Triangular Atlantic Race with stops at Cape Town and Rio de Janeiro, ending at Portsmouth.

It was not long after this race that Eric first came up with the idea of building another revolutionary trimaran capable of very high speeds by the use of hydrofoils to lift the hulls above the waves. This was planned to be his entry for the 1976 OSTAR. Tabarly discussed the idea with aeronautical engineers at the Dassault aeroplane company but they said the idea would not work with the materials then available to them. Carbon fibre and the like lay in the future. It was, however, thought possible to use foils to give added lift to the floats, which could then be kept much smaller, saving weight and drag.

Plans were drawn up for a foil-assisted aluminium trimaran but no builder could be found to build it in time, not even the

French Navy. Tabarly therefore decided to enter the OSTAR with his old *Pen Duick VI* which, as we have seen, was a huge vessel normally sailed by a crew of 12. Despite having sailed the boat for many thousands of miles, the race organisers still insisted that Tabarly undertook a mandatory solo 500 mile qualifying trip.

So in May 1976 Tabarly was back in Millbay Dock, twelve years after his initial triumph which had changed his life. He felt ready for the challenge and had an army of helpers to prepare the huge boat including, many complained, half the French Navy. Not many thought that Tabarly would be able to handle *Pen Duick VI* on his own, but the same was also said of some of his competitors, particularly two of his protégées. One was Alain Colas with his enormous 238-foot *Club Mediterranee* and the other was Yvon Fauconnier, with the 120-foot three-masted schooner originally conceived by Jean Eves Terlain and now renamed *ITT Oceanic*. Terlain himself was now sailing *Kriter III*, Robin Knox-Johnston's old 70-foot catamaran, previously called *British Oxygen*.

This was to be Tabarly's toughest race. Soon after the start on 5 June he took the lead. On 11 June a deep depression swept across the fleet. At the same time another low was brewing up over New England. This deepened and, by the end of the next day, was right in the middle of the Atlantic, giving storm force head winds to all competitors, other than those few who had headed south. Fauconnier on the huge *ITT Oceanic* broke an arm and tore his sails. Terlain's catamaran *Kriter III* began to break up and sink. A Russian tug went to their rescue, picking up Terlain and towing *ITT Oceanic* into St John's in Newfoundland. There were numerous other casualties, amongst them Angus Primrose in *Demon Demo* who was rolled through 360 degrees and lost his mast. Alain Colas on the mighty *Club Mediterranee* was beset by halyard problems and torn sails. He also put into St John's to repair the damage. This was probably the storm in which *Three Cheers* and Mike McMullen were lost.

Throughout all this mayhem there was silence from Tabarly. In the early hours of 29 June he crossed the finishing line and then sailed the 73 foot yacht all the way into the marina at Goat Island and moored up before anyone else was awake or knew of his arrival. He was first in a time of 23 days and 20 hours.

Tabarly spoke after the race of facing 50 knot headwinds soon after the start, of his self-steering gear failing to work, leading to hour after hour at the wheel in appalling conditions. He faced a succession of four gales one after another. During the fourth, with winds of over 60 knots he decided to head south to try to get some kinder weather. He arrived utterly exhausted and a photograph taken soon after his arrival shows him sitting wearily on the deck of his boat the demands of the race etched clearly on his haggard face and sunken eyes. He said afterwards that when he was told he was first he so wasted he even lacked the energy for 'exuberance in a time of victory.'

The race had been one of the most demanding ever and it was an achievement for this small man to have sailed his huge and heavy yacht through such atrocious weather to beat all the competition. A few days later he flew to New York and then boarded an Air France flight to Paris. There he found himself in front of TV cameras and the press and was obliged to parade along the Champs-Elysée cheered by an enthusiastic crowd. Tabarly tried to get out of this demonstration but was persuaded to go along with it as he had become the centre of attention for thousands of admirers.

This was really the end of Tabarly's successful racing career. Years passed and he continued to sail *Pen Duick VI* around the world's oceans covering more than three hundred thousand miles and seven oceans. There were however to be no more *Pen Duicks*. He campaigned several other boats but never had the same successes and it appeared as if his heart was not really in it any longer. Once the *Pen Duick* name went, some of the vitality and drive seemed to go from Tabarly. Maybe it was just that he was getting old.

In the years to come he did eventually build his 60-foot foil as-sisted trimaran, giving it the name *Paul Ricard*, after the sponsors who paid for it. He planned to race it in the 1980 OSTAR but he was forced to withdraw due to an old skiing injury. The race organisers did not allow Tabarly to hand the boat over to Marc Pajot, one of his many protégés. After much argument with the Race Committee it was agreed that Pajot could take part in the race, but not as an official entrant. Tabarly did sail *Paul Ricard* in the next OSTAR in 1984 and came in fourth in a time of 16 days and 14 hours. He never warmed to or spoke much of this boat, which went through many alterations, was never very suc-cessful and was a handful to sail.

Tabarly then obtained sponsorship from Cote d'Or, the Belgian chocolate manufacturers, and had a 25 metre maxi yacht built for the 1985/6 Whitbread Round the World Race in which they finished a poor tenth out of thirteen finishers. The next year, not having sufficient funds to build a new boat, Tabarly took his old *Paul Ricard* trimaran discarded all but the main hull and built two new crossbeams with longer floats and foils. Re-branded *Cote d'Or II*, Tabarly entered her for the 1986

Route de Rhum from France to Guadeloupe. When nearing the finish, a large part of one of the floats broke off, the boat nearly capsized and Tabarly had to retire. Tabarly's brother, Patrick, who was sailing nearby on board *Pen Duick VI* located the broken part of the float and towed it in to harbour.

In 1987 Tabarly and Patrick entered *Cote d'Or II* for the La Baule-Dakar Two Handed Race. They capsized 60 miles from Madeira but were quickly rescued.

In 1989, at the age of 58, Tabarly took part in the two handed 'Transat en Double' a two handed race from Lorient in France, round Bermuda and back to France without stopping. His boat was a new generation trimaran called *Bottin Enterprise* and his crew was Jean Lecam (who later became a successful skipper himself). They had a good first outward leg and were leading on the way home when they capsized, probably as a result of Tabarly pushing the boat too hard. They were travelling very fast with a large spinnaker set and Tabarly, who had been at the helm for a long time, was flagging. Jean Lecam was below decks on the radio. As the boat reared up on one float and went over, Tabarly was thrown out about thirty feet above the sea and fractured his collar bone. He managed to swim back to the upturned hull and climb back on board. Inside, Lecam got out via an escape hatch in the stern. For some six hours they sat on the upturned hull until a cargo ship arrived and picked them up.

Tabarly admitted afterwards that this was the only time he had really been frightened at sea as it all happened so quickly and was something over which he had no control. He raced little after that and in his early sixties decided to retire.

Up until that time Tabarly had had no real family life. He lived for his sailing, devoting himself full time to his boats and racing. However, in 1976 he met a girl, Jacqueline, on a friend's boat. For eight years they continued to see each other and finally got married in Brittany in 1984. They bought a house there, an old barn overlooking a river. This was the first house Tabarly had ever owned. Later they had a daughter, Marie.

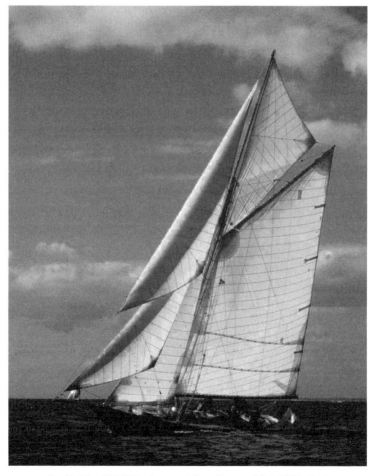

Pen Duick which Tabarly owned from the age of 21 till his death

Often thereafter Tabarly would hole up in his study with his books, pictures, boat models and magazines reminding him of his life as a sailor and remembering his various boats. Nearest to his heart, was the first *Pen Duick*. Tabarly spent much time every winter restoring and maintaining her and readying her for her centenary year in 1998.

Before that event, in 1989 Tabarly was invited to attend a major maritime festival to be held at Rouen on the River Seine. Tabarly refused the invitation as he did not have enough money to get *Pen Duick* seaworthy for such a trip. When told of this, the Mayor of Rouen announced that they had to have Tabarly and that the city would advance whatever money was needed. *Pen Duick* attended the festival and was one of the major attractions.

In 1998 a group of yachtsmen, all of whom owned yachts designed and built by William Fife III, the legendary Scottish yacht designer and builder, decided to hold the first ever regatta and re-union of Fife boats. This was to be held on the Firth of Clyde in Scotland, near the original boatyard at Fairlie where the boats had been built. It was pure coincidence that 1998 also happened to be the centenary year of the launch of *Pen Duick*. Hearing of the regatta, Tabarly immediately decided to take his beloved boat to Scotland to attend this gathering.

Tabarly assembled a crew to help him sail to Scotland. They were Erwan Quenere, a well-known French photographer, Lieutenant Jacques Rebec, an old skiing friend of Tabarly, and Antoine Costa and his wife, Candida. They were hardly a racing crew but were rather friends on a cruise, which was how Tabarly now preferred to sail.

By early June they were at Newlyn, a small Cornish fishing port, where they were held up for several days by northerly gales. They were sailing north in company with another Fife, the Swedish *Magda IV*, having sailed together from Benodet in Brittany, where they had just celebrated *Pen Duick*'s centenary.

The northerly gales had ceased by Friday 12 June and the forecast was favourable with winds backing to the south. No mention was made of bad weather. The two boats left harbour in the late morning, having agreed to make radio contact every three hours.

In Tabarly's customary manner, *Pen Duick* soon set full sail, which meant three jibs, a large gaff mainsail and a jackyard topsail. *Magda IV* left under reduced sail and soon fell behind. *Pen Duick* passed Land's End in the early afternoon and ran into a large swell left over from the northerly gales. As they progressed conditions got more difficult. The wind had now gone round to the south, blowing strongly against this swell kicking up a nasty short chop with breaking seas. *Pen Duick* has very low freeboard and the seas were beginning to break over her decks. Tabarly decided to shorten sail.

As to what happened next it must be appreciated that *Pen Duick* had no winches, no pulpit, no guardrails or jackstays and, as far as is known, Tabarly never wore a life jacket or safety harness. His boats never carried any. Tabarly once said he would prefer to spend an hour in the water rather than be tied on with a harness.

Tabarly went forward to the mast and took in one reef and then two as the wind continued to increase. Around midnight the boat was still over canvassed with just a double reefed mainsail and a small jib. The seas were growing bigger and *Pen Duick* was being repeatedly struck by squalls bringing with them thick rain and zero visibility. The seas were three to four metres high over which she was surging at some nine knots, rolling from rail to rail with the wind dead aft.

Eric now decided to replace the mainsail with a storm trysail. Whilst a difficult manoeuvre, it was something Tabarly had done thousands of times before. It involved hauling in the main boom and sheeting it in hard to the centreline, then the gaff's peak and throat halyards had to be lowered whilst the crew bundled in the sail quickly to prevent it being blown off into the water. At the same time the gaff had to be secured and lashed down to prevent the boat's rolling setting it swinging wildly from side to side around the heads of the crew. Then the trysail could be bent on and hoisted.

It was pitch dark and Tabarly asked Erwan Quemere to take the helm. Erwan, a good sailor, asked Tabarly if he should turn the boat head to wind. Tabarly told him to stay as he was. Erwan, not wishing to argue with Tabarly, concentrated on keeping *Pen Duick* on course dead down wind.

Antoine Costa and Jacques Rebec went forward to the mast and uncleated the two halyards and began to lower the gaff's peak and throat. Costa's wife remained in the cockpit. Then Antoine moved further aft to help gather in the sail. Tabarly was further aft still standing on the deck with his chest leaning against the boom fighting furiously with the sail. The gaff was lowered onto the now stowed sail and all that was needed was for a lashing to be passed around the gaff and boom to make it fast.

At that moment *Pen Duick* rolled violently and the gaff swung out to starboard only to swing back hitting Tabarly full in the chest. He lost his footing and was thrown backwards overboard into the sea.

Tabarly began to drift away into the darkness. The crew threw life buoys into the sea and launched red parachute rockets. They could not see the lights of any ships in the vicinity and they knew that the only radio on board, a hand held VHF, would not be heard on the nearest land. They were 80 miles north of Land's End and 35 miles off the South Wales coast.

In a state of shock, the crew lowered the small jib, started the boat's small auxiliary engine, an 18 HP Volvo diesel with a small two-bladed propeller, and tried to motor back upwind to where they thought Tabarly might be. They made little progress. The engine was only good for manoeuvring in harbour (Tabarly liked to do everything under sail). It took them over three hours to get back to where they thought Tabarly had gone overboard but there was no sign of him. After a few hours searching they decided to head for land hoping to meet a ship or fishing boat. As dawn approached the wind and sea died down and it was an extremely distressed and traumatised crew who motored *Pen Duick* toward the Welsh coast.

At daybreak they saw a large racing yacht heading toward them. They let off a red flare and the yacht closed with them. The boat was the Maxi racing yacht *Longobarda* owned by property magnate Mike Slade on its way to Ireland. The battery in *Pen Duick*'s VHF was flat and *Longobarda* had to get close alongside to hear what the crew were shouting. *Longobarda* contacted the Milford Haven Coastguard at seven o'clock. An RAF helicopter and the Angle lifeboat were ordered to the scene where several other ships, including a Royal Navy minesweeper, joined in the search. As soon as news that Tabarly was missing reached France, a French military aeroplane arrived and patrolled until nightfall but nothing was found.

The Angle lifeboat accompanied *Pen Duick* into Milford Haven. The crew were in a state of shock. Erwan Quemere recalled that it had been a dream to sail from Benodet with Tabarly but that the dream had turned into a nightmare. Afterwards some people said the crew were too inexperienced and that they should have been able to rescue him. This is unfair criticism and what happened could have happened to anyone. *Pen Duick* was an old boat, with no winches and all sail handling was hard work and took time. The engine was not powerful enough to work to windward under those conditions and once Tabarly had gone overboard it would only be pure chance that they were ever going to find and retrieve him.

Another Fife yacht on its way to the Clyde, the *Kentra*, heard these events on the radio and put into Milford Haven to help the crew of *Pen Duick*. Tabarly in the past had often helmed *Kentra* in races in the Mediterranean. *Magda IV* joined them and all three boats sailed north together to attend the regatta. This was a sober affair which became a gesture of homage to France's greatest ever sailor.

Tabarly's body was found 37 days later on 20 July 1998 by a fishing trawler and flown back to France, where he was given a hero's funeral and he was buried in Brittany.

Soon after his death the Association Eric Tabarly was formed with the objects of keeping Tabarly's legacy alive and of ensuring that the various *Pen Duick* yachts were kept and maintained as seagoing vessels for all time. For many years, Jacqueline Tabarly was the Association's President.

Chapter 11

The Extraordinary Life and Last Voyage of Philip Walwyn on board his 12 Metre Yacht *Kate* (2015)

At the beginning of 1974 a young naval architect and yacht builder, Andrew Simpson, launched his latest creation, a sleek 35-foot trimaran. She had long, low and narrow hulls and a substantial beam. She was a refinement of a design he had used several times before. She was called *Whisky Jack* and he painted her bright primrose yellow. One innovation on her was that she had a daggerboard in each float rather than a single centreboard in the main hull. These were asymmetric and aerofoil in section which created lift when sailing fast and they could be said to be one of the first tentative examples of the foils now fitted to the latest America's Cup machines flying at over 30 knots.

Andrew had built *Whisky Jack* with the intention of taking part in the 1974 Round Britain and Ireland Race. However, at the time of her launch, Britain was in the depths of an economic crisis, facing the miners' strike and power cuts. The then Prime Minister, Ted Heath, introduced the Three Day Week on 1 January 1974. The economic situation badly affected Andrew Simpson's business and orders dried up.

He decided there was no future for him in England and that he would emigrate to the USA and try his luck there. He cancelled his entry in the race, loaded his belongings onto *Whisky*

Jack and he and his wife set off to sail across the Atlantic to Galveston in Texas, where a prospective partner for his new business waited. Everything was basic and simple on board the trimaran. They had no electricity and they carried only paraffin navigation lamps (legal then, but not now). They had no electronic navigation instruments or engine. The trip was successful, the boat proved to be seaworthy and fast and they started anew in the USA.

The next year a young Philip Walwyn, then aged 28, travelled from his home on the island of St Kitts in the West Indies to Galveston to buy *Whisky Jack* and sail her back to his home. This started Philip's sailing career. For the next few years he sailed the trimaran throughout the Caribbean and took part in three editions of the Saint Maarten Tradewinds Race, then the only ocean race in the West Indies. The race was over an 800-mile course from the island of St Maarten round Martinique and back. Philip won this race in *Whisky Jack* in 1975.

In the spring of 1978 Philip and his fiancée, Frances Tate, sailed *Whisky Jack* to England, stopping at Bermuda on the way. They arrived in Plymouth just in time to enter that year's Round Britain and Ireland Race starting on 8 July. I too was taking part in that race, on board another trimaran called *Heretic*, sailing with Exeter policeman Peter Phillips. I had not seen Philip Walwyn since we were childhood friends and it was the first time I had ever seen *Whisky Jack*.

*

Philip was born in 1947, 4 years after me. His father was an army officer and the family spent the summer months in their house alongside the yacht harbour at Birdham Pool outside Chichester in West Sussex. The winters were spent on their sugar plantation on the island of St Kitts in the West Indies.

I first met the Walwyns in the late 1950s, when I used to spend my holidays on board my father's boat berthed in Birdham Pool. (It was also there that I first met Peter Tangvald – see Chapter 9.) I and my sister had a Firefly dinghy, as did Philip, and we, along with Philip's two sisters, Susan and Jill, spent our summers messing about in boats, racing dinghies and crewing on other people's yachts in and around Chichester harbour. I and my sister, coming from an impoverished naval family, were insanely jealous of the Walwyn's lifestyle. For a short while Susan became my first teenage girlfriend and we wrote letters to each other from our boarding schools, hers on pink scented notepaper.

Whilst growing up Philip saw little of his father, who was then an army Colonel largely serving abroad in Aden and Cyprus. During the Second World War he had served with distinction in the British army, being awarded the Military Cross and the Distinguished Service Order. He served in Kenya in the King's African Rifles and later in Egypt and Burma. I recall Philip's father as a small brusque man with a neat military moustache and a somewhat intimidating manner.

As Philip grew up he formed a deep and abiding interest in sailing yachts, mostly gained from watching the shipwrights at Birdham Pool and Itchenor building and repairing wooden yachts in the traditional manner. Philip's father bought him a series of racing dinghies - a Cadet, a Firefly and then a 14 Foot International, all of which Philip raced successfully.

Philip hated his preparatory school in Fernhurst in Sussex and was miserable at his public school, Wellington College, where he was sent as his father was adamant that Philip should follow him into the Army, a career for which Philip could not have been less well suited. On leaving Wellington, Philip wanted to become an apprentice to a naval architect with a view to becoming a yacht designer. His father thought otherwise and Philip was enrolled into the Royal Military Academy at Sandhurst. Life at Sandhurst did not suit Philip at all and, after he had been there for only a short period, he was told he was 'idle, blasé and indifferent.' He decided to leave (or he may have been asked to leave).

Philip was sent next to the Royal Agricultural College at Cirencester with a view to him joining his father, now retired from the Army, in running the family's sugar estates at St Rawlins on the island of St Kitts. The Walwyn family had inherited these estates some years previously. On graduating from Cirencester Philip left England for good to live in the Caribbean.

He lived and worked there helping his father run the estates until 1974, when the newly independent government of St Kitts and Nevis nationalised all the sugar plantations on the islands and took most of the land at St Rawlins. The Walwyns were left with just a few acres, their house called the Mount Pleasant Plantation House, and the old sugar factory buildings. Philip started and operated a market garden and ran a beef herd on what land was left to them, from where he supplied local hotels and restaurants.

It was by pure chance that one year the Rockefeller family from New York were staying at the Nesbit Plantation Hotel, a privately owned resort on the island of Nevis, which was that year being managed by Philip's father and mother. This hotel had at one time been the house of Fanny Nesbit who married Horatio Nelson and became Lady Nelson. Following a visit by

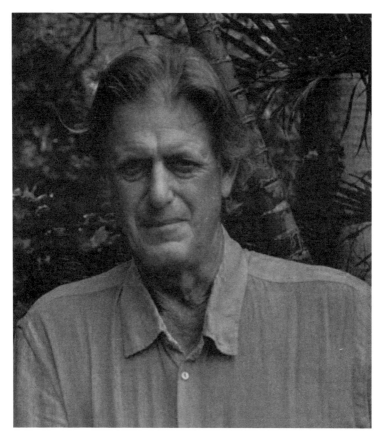

Philip Walwyn

the Rockefeller party to the Walwyn's property on St Kitts, one of them suggested that the Mount Pleasant Plantation House should be turned into a hotel. Philip and his father took up this suggestion and the Rawlins Plantation Hotel, as they called it, soon became one of the best known and exclusive resorts of its type in the Caribbean. The success of this gave Philip the financial resources to take up serious blue water sailing.

In 1975 Philip travelled to Galveston and bought *Whisky Jack*.
In 1979 Philip founded a boat building business on St Kitts, which built a number of multihulls between 40 and 75 feet, most designed by the Caribbean naval architect, Peter Spronk. These included a 45-foot Spronk catamaran which Philip built for himself in 1981, calling it *Sky Jack*. In this he crossed the Atlantic four times. He first bought her over to Europe in 1981 for the TWOSTAR, crewed by his wife, Frances. They put up a very good performance in what was a heavy weather race, coming in fourth in their class and fifteenth overall. As recounted in Chapter 8, the race was won by Chay Blyth and Rob James in their 65-foot *Brittany Ferries GB*.

Philip and Frances were back in Europe for the next Round Britain and Ireland Race in 1982. This time they won their class and were tenth overall out of 69 finishers. This race was won by Rob and Naomi James in *Colt Cars GB*. After this race, they sailed *Sky Jack* to St Malo from where Philip raced her alone to Guadeloupe in the French race, the Route de Rhum. Philip, sailing one of the smallest boats, finished in the middle of the fleet. He put up the fastest time for the final 'sprint' to the finish line at Guadeloupe.

Next in 1984 Philip built a much larger Spronk catamaran, the 75-foot *Spirit of St Kitts*, in which Philip sailed six times across the Atlantic, one time solo. In 1984 he took part in a 3,000-mile race organised by the French from Quebec to St Malo and in 1986 entered her into the two-handed Carlsberg Transatlantic Race, crewed again with his wife. Unfortunately, during a period of heavy weather, the boat developed leaks in both hulls. They were forced to retire, whereupon they sailed straight home to St Kitts.

After these adventures Philip turned his back on multihulls and built, sailed and raced conventional single hulled yachts for the rest of his life. Part of the reason would have been the ever increasing cost of building and campaigning multihulls for long distance racing. Huge sums of money were now involved, together with a creeping professionalism and the need for a large shore team, none of which would have sat well with Philip's idiosyncratic character.

Philip next turned his inventive hands to the rarefied, exclusive and expensive sport of racing International 6 Metre yachts. These are baby sisters to the 12 Metre yachts which were then being used for racing in the America's Cup, a race which Great Britain inaugurated but has never won. The 6 Metre yacht class is very old but was experiencing a renaissance at the time with many new boats being built, all equipped with the latest high-tech sails and gear. They are long, narrow, extremely elegant and beautiful boats and are raced on inshore courses all over the world. Many of the older pre-Second World War boats have been re-built or refurbished and now race alongside their modern high-tech versions, giving close and extremely competitive racing.

In 1986, following his last multihull race, Philip commissioned Ian Howlett to design, and the Elephant Boatyard to build, a new 6 Metre to be named *St Kitts*. The Elephant Boatyard, run by Tom Richardson, lies on a bend of the river Hamble squeezed onto a small piece of land between the river and a railway line and is next to the famous sailors' pub, the Jolly Sailor. The yard was at that time known to millions of television viewers as it was used as the set for the popular TV series *Howards Way* which ran on BBC TV for many years. The Elephant had been founded by Tom's father Mike Richardson at the end of the Second World War and had carved out a niche for itself in maintaining old classic wooden boats and in building high quality new ones. *HMS Elephant*, Nelson's flagship at the Battle of Copenhagen, had been built on the site of the boatyard, hence its name.

Upon completion of *St Kitts* Philip had her shipped to Seawanaka in Oyster Bay, New York for the 1986 6 Metre World Championships. They finished in eighth place – a considerable achievement for a new and untried boat. This was a first attempt by Philip in racing against some of the best sailors in the world, on yachts which are notoriously difficult to sail well.

In 1988 Philip and *St Kitts* were back in England. First they won the 6 Metre British Championships run by the Royal Yacht Squadron in Cowes on the Isle of Wight. They then entered the 6 Metre European Championships, held at Falmouth in Cornwall. They won this too, becoming the first British boat ever to win this event. After that Philip put *St Kitts* up for sale but had no takers. He shipped her to the Caribbean, where he inaugurated a 6 Metre regatta to take place in St Kitts and Nevis. For this event Philip built, at his home, a sister ship which he called *St Kitts II* (now sold and called *Wildcat II*). A number of 'Sixes' took part in the first of these regattas and Philip came in sixth in the original *St Kitts*. Soon after this he sold both of his 6 Metres.

Some years later later Philip bought yet another 6 Metre from Port Huron in the USA. She was called *Circe II* and Philip renamed her *St Kitts III*. In order to qualify for the Antigua Classic Regattas, he had to raise the gunwhales by six inches and he laid a new deck. Philip related that he won this event, but was subsequently disqualified due, he maintained, to official handicapping errors. The yacht was subsequently shipped back to the

Elephant Boatyard and sold.

Wanting a return to short-handed long distance racing, in 1988 Philip decided to build a very radical state of the art 40-foot carbon fibre monohull racing yacht, with an all carbon-fibre swing rig and unstayed mast. She was designed by Ian Howlett and built at Bembridge on the Isle of Wight. Like all his boats, he had her and her mast painted his trademark bright yellow. After her launch he sailed the boat solo across the Atlantic home to St Kitts, where he altered the fixed keel to a canting keel. Now commonplace on racing yachts, this is believed to have been the first time such a device was tried out on an ocean racing yacht. They have proved to be problematical devices but give much added stability, without increasing weight. They allow yachts to carry a much larger sail area. The next year he sailed, again solo, from St Kitts to Plymouth but he found the boat extremely uncomfortable, hard to handle and the rig almost impossible to get to work properly. A year later he attempted another solo transatlantic voyage but after two days out from Plymouth, with everything going wrong, he was washed overboard by a freak wave in a force 10 storm. This time he was wearing a safety harness and Philip recalled how he was towed alongside the hull in mountainous seas for some ten minutes. He really believed he was going to drown. Luckily a wave washed him back over the guardrails onto the deck. Concussed, battered and bruised, not knowing whether he had broken anything, he turned back to Plymouth.

On arrival and still suffering from the after effects of concussion, Philip was interviewed on a local television station when he declared that he would sell the boat to the first person to give him a pound. Later someone did hand him a £1 note and the man and boat have never been seen again.

Philip retired somewhat hurt to the Caribbean. This was Philip's last attempt at competitive ocean racing. He spent the next few years in and around St Kitts and his St Rawlins hotel. During this period his marriage to Frances ended in divorce and in 1992 he married the artist Kate Spencer.

In 1995 he built a 30 foot very fast American-designed 'Cigarette' power boat equipped with twin 250 HP Yamaha outboards and minimal accommodation. She was, of course, painted bright yellow. In this he cruised (at a very high speed) through the Caribbean to Florida, up through the east coast of the USA on the intra-coastal waterway, along the St John's River and up to New York then onward to Cape Cod and finally to Kennebunkport in Maine. Philip had intended to continue up to Canada, then down the St Lawrence Seaway into the Great Lakes and finally down the Mississippi River to New Orleans, the Gulf of Mexico and home to St Kitts. He ran out of time and had the boat shipped home to St Kitts.

A year later Philip bought a classic 91-foot wooden motor yacht called *Tiger* which had been built on the river Clyde in Scotland in 1927. Philip rescued her from the mangrove swamps at English Harbour in Antigua where she had lain rotting away for many years, having been abandoned by her then owner, an American millionaire rancher from Oregon. Philip had *Tiger* towed the 50 miles from Antigua to St Kitts where she just passed through a narrow channel between coral reefs to get into Dieppe Bay, close to Philip's home. There he stripped out the former owner's melamine covered plywood and vinyl 'caravan style' interior, complete with what Philip described as 'a psychedelic paint job.' He restored her to her former glory as a gentleman's yacht, complete with a fine saloon and library furnished with 18th century mahogany furniture. Philip dismantled the original twin Gardner engines, which had been ruined by salt water, and installed two re-conditioned Gardner diesels shipped out from England.

Philip and his wife Kate cruised in her twice to Venezuela and once to Cuba. On the return journey, when 150 miles south of Cuba, they ran into some rough weather. *Tiger* sprung a plank and began to leak badly. Philip arranged by radio telephone for a large volume pump to be flown up from St Kitts on board a Falcon 4 private jet which proceeded to parachute the pump into the sea. Philip intended to recover the pump with his inflatable RIB dinghy which he was towing behind *Tiger*. However, in rough seas this whole attempt was unsuccessful.

Ultimately Philip and Kate were rescued by a large heavily armed US Coastguard Drug Patrol vessel, the crew of which put some powerful pumps on board *Tiger*, attached a tow-line and tried to tow her back to Cuba. However, the weather worsened and the tow became impractical.

Rather than leave the boat half afloat and in Philip's words 'to put her out of her misery' he famously asked the Coastguard to fire on the stricken boat and sink her. This they did with heavy machine gun fire. Poor *Tiger* took a long time to sink and it was a sad demise for a ship that had once served as a British Royal Navy patrol ship during World War II as *HMS Tiger*.

Back on dry land Philip set about getting together a team of boat builders to help him build his last boat. This was a First Rule International 12 Metre yacht and was built to the same 1908 lines as a famous 12 Metre called *Javotte*, designed by the esteemed Victorian yacht designer Alfred Mylne. When completed the new 12 Metre was one of the most striking and head-turning boats to have been built in recent years, only spoilt, according to many people, by her bright yellow colour which everyone hated. "It annoys a lot of people which is rather satisfying," Philip was reported as saying. Later he painted her black.

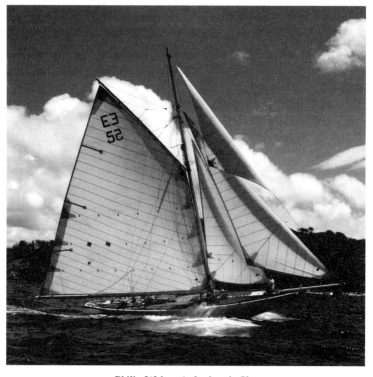

Philip Walwyn's final yacht Kate

The boat named *Kate*, after Philip's wife, was over 23 metres from the tip of her bowsprit to the end of her boom, 19 metres on deck with a beam of 3.45 metres and a depth of 2.30 metres. She was built next to Philip's house on St Kitts and transported over land to be launched. The hull was built of strip pine planking, sheathed in glass cloth and epoxy, with an 11-ton lead keel. She had no engine, no tanks and, apart from a masthead navigation light, no electrics. The below deck accommodation was kept simple and basic. In 2007 Philip said in an interview, "The drum I like beating is this thing called simplicity. It's much more difficult but much more rewarding." *Kate* boasts a piece of the original *Javotte*. On hearing of the project, the son of the last owner sent Philip one of *Javotte*'s bronze fairleads.

Originally built as a gaff cutter with a jackyard topsail, Philip later converted her to ketch rig, retaining the gaff mainsail. This made her easier to handle short- or single-handed. Later still, and for his last single-handed voyage from St Kitts to England, Philip replaced the gaff mainsail with a Bermudan one.

For several years Philip sailed and raced *Kate* all over the Caribbean and had four firsts out of ten races in regattas at St Maarten, St Bart's, the British Virgin Islands and Antigua.

In 2014 Philip decided to bring *Kate* over to Europe and, probably because he could not find any suitable crew to undertake such a long voyage, he set out to sail her single-handed. This was probably the first time anyone had tried to cross the Atlantic alone on a 12 Metre. But he was an extremely competent and experienced sailor and he made appropriate and sensible changes to the rig. He dispensed with the main boom and used a small loose-footed mainsail. He put a permanent reef in the gaff-rigged mizzen so as to raise the boom, allowing for a wind vane self-steering gear to be set. He still had no engine but installed two solar panels to charge the batteries to power the navigation lights and a few instruments. He had a hand held GPS receiver, a VHF radio and a satellite phone. This was to be his seventeenth transatlantic crossing, on six of which he had been alone.

Philip planned to have an engine fitted to *Kate* in England and then to take her south to the Mediterranean, maybe to be sold, so that he could start on his next project, which he spoke about before he left. This was to build an even larger yacht – a replica of the 40-metre Alfred Mylne designed *Octavia*, built in 1910 to the International 19 Metre rule. Philip said he wanted to build a 'better looking version' in wood and epoxy, to rival the current darling of the Mediterranean classic super yacht circuit, the huge *Mariquita*.

Philip and *Kate* set off from St Kitts on 6 June 2014, intending to sail straight to the Azores. However, he met with light contrary winds for most of the early part of the voyage and was pushed further north than he intended. On 17 June he sent a message saying that he now planned to head for Nova Scotia rather than the Azores. He was 150 miles south of Bermuda and said 'Becalmed - Reading War and Peace.' On 19 June he sent a further message 'Still becalmed – gone back 5 miles from yesterday's position.' On 22 June he said he had some breeze and was 600 miles from Lunenburg in Nova Scotia. On 25 June he had 300 miles to go. He arrived at Lunenburg on 1 July and left *Kate* there for the winter.

In the spring of 2015 Philip set sail, again single-handed, from Nova Scotia planning to make for the Azores and then England. A week out he encountered a severe storm which wiped out his self-steering gear; Philip was unable to repair it at sea. He arrived off Horta in the Azores in darkness and hove to for the night. He was very tired on arrival the next morning. His wife, Kate, flew over from the Caribbean and they spent a week together exploring the islands. Philip managed to repair his self-steering gear but soon after he left for England he ran into another gale, which once again demolished it. Philip continued steering by hand making good progress. On 1 August 2015 he had 300 miles to go. Philip approached the Scilly Isles on the night of 2 August. Early the next morning he contacted his sister Susan and reported that he had spent the night dodging shipping and was exhausted. He contacted her again later that day, when he was off the Lizard and asked Susan to meet him in Falmouth. Susan asked him what he would like for lunch – "oh a salad please," Philip said.

Susan heard nothing more until she received a message at around two o'clock from Philip's wife, Kate, to say that *Kate* had been seen going round in circles with all its sails set off Coverack Cove with no one on board. Susan contacted the Falmouth Coastguard who told her there was a major sea search operation being conducted by the Air Sea Rescue Service at Culdrose.

The crew of a private yacht, which was passing on its way home from a cruise in Brittany, joined in the search and moved to a point close to Black Head. They started a zig-zag search and at around five o'clock they saw something in the water which turned out to be a person lying face down very close into the rocks. The yacht motored up to the casualty, who was not wearing a lifejacket or a safety harness. The crew could not get hold of anything with which to lift the body out of the water, nor could they get a rope around it. All they could do was hold onto it and motor slowly out into deeper water. They called the Coastguard and within a few minutes a helicopter arrived and recovered the body. It was indeed Philip, who was still alive but had been in the water for some four to five hours. The helicopter took him ashore. As it landed at the Royal Cornwall Hospital at

Treliske, Philip had a massive heart attack and died.

He was only 10 miles from his destination when he fell overboard having sailed his 12 Metre racing yacht single-handed across the Atlantic, most of the way without any form of self-steering.

Susan said later that this was to have been Philip's last transatlantic crossing. Philip's widow Kate thinks that Philip, who had suffered health problems for some time, probably had a heart attack on board and then fell overboard.

Some years previously Philip was asked why he had built *Kate*. He replied that it was just another mad dream and said "most people live lives of quiet desperation and die with the song still in them."

Kate, his widow, said of him, "Philip grew angry with himself on land. He was a heavy man but he turned into a ballerina once on a boat." What more can one say about a great sailor and a man loved by all those with whom he came into contact. He will be sorely missed by his family and friends.

Kate was brought into Falmouth, lifted ashore and put up for sale. She has now been sold to a Swedish hi-tech Silicon Valley magnate, Anders Swahn, who had her transported by road to Portugal. After a major re-fit, she will be sailed to a new home in California.

Afterword

The impetuosity of youth combined with the fatalistic attitude of an 80-year-old willing to accept his end at sea in the Antarctic. Money pressures destroying long-held dreams and a refusal to accept reality. A determination to overcome the trauma of the loss of a beloved partner. Caught out in unexpected appalling weather conditions with an inexperienced crew. Sheer bad luck leading to a fatal fall overboard. Corrosion on an old boat causing it to break up and sink. A sudden disabling heart attack whilst nearing land.

Each of these factors could explain the deaths recounted herein. Perhaps a major factor might also be over-familiarity with the sea which inevitably comes after sailing the world's oceans year after year, combined with increasing age and infirmity.

There is no single answer which can explain the tragedies described here. Ages range from 25 (Simon Richardson) to 80 (Bill Tilman). The youngest and the oldest were lost together on the same boat in the South Atlantic. Six others were in their thirties, two in their fifties (Frank Davison and Angus Primrose) and three in their sixties (Eric Tabarly and Peter Tangvald were both 67 and Philip Walwyn was 68).

One factor, which is common to nearly all the tragedies is the lack of life jackets or safety harnesses. This is a controversial area, complicated by the fact that the use of such aids was far less frequent in the past than it is today. A number of the sailors were well known for their abhorrence of the use of such devices. Tabarly never used them and famously said that he would prefer to spend a few hours in the water rather than to be dragged along by a still moving boat. Rob James was not wearing either a life jacket or a safety harness. Had he donned a harness, he might not have gone over the side and had he worn a life jacket he may have survived the time he was in the water. Philip Walwyn was not a believer in them but he was wearing one on the occasion when he was washed overboard from his small monohull in the north Atlantic. This probably saved him. He was not, however, wearing a life jacket or safety harness when found after he had fallen overboard from *Kate*, at the end of his last voyage.

Mike McMullen after his tumble from the foredeck of *Three Cheers* in the Round Britain Race, which nearly drowned him, said that on *Three Cheers* they wore safety harnesses or life jackets when they thought 'conditions warranted it.' However, he did admit that the incident was a salutary lesson and he would think more carefully about their use in the future.

Surprisingly Tilman, who never thought much about his or his crew's safety and never took on his long ocean voyages any form of safety equipment – no flares, no life jackets and no life rafts – did comment on the low freeboard and lack of guardrails or life lines on *En Avant*'s wide deck. However, this may have been more an expression of his disgust at finding it difficult at his age to propel himself around the decks rather than a concern for the crew's safety. It is not known what sort of safety equipment *En Avant* carried, but in the circumstances none would have been of much use if, as is supposed, the boat turned turtle and sank quickly.

Lack of money and a desire to carry on regardless was a feature of several of the voyages. Everything on *En Avant* was done on the cheap. Maybe because of the cost, or more likely as a result of Simon's somewhat arrogant and over confident belief in his own ability, no professional advice was sought on the conversion or on the quality of the work carried out. No qualified surveyor would ever have allowed a ballast keel to be added to an old steel hull merely by the welding of some steel plates to the bottom without some well thought-out through-hull bolting, especially if the hollow box keel was later to be filled with lead or iron ballast. The lack of any such ballast would have left *En Avant* extremely vulnerable and tender and this most probably contributed to her loss.

None of this concerned Simon, who was maybe seduced by an oft quoted remark of Tilman. When asked how someone could get on an expedition to get to the Himalayas, Tilman merely said "Just put on your boots and go." One of Tilman's biographers, Tim Madge, suggests that Tilman did Simon no service when the old man suggested that "any worthwhile exploration could be planned on the back of an envelope." Simon was not an experienced sailor. He had crewed on a few delivery trips around northern Europe and, apart from one trip to Greenland as part of Tilman's crew on board *Baroque*, he had no experience of sailing in high latitudes. He did have Tilman on board with all his experience of polar waters, but Tilman took no part in the handling of what he called 'this steel monster.' He said poignantly in a letter sent from Rio to a friend in England 'I don't know why I am here.' To back this up there are two photographs of the old man on board *En Avant*, one taken as they left Southampton, showing Tilman staring backwards at the passing water lost in his own thoughts. The other was taken somewhere near the equator in the boat's cabin on the occasion of Simon's 25th birthday. It shows a haggard Tilman looking quizzically and somewhat out of place as Simon blows out candles on a cake whilst the crew, who are obviously enjoying themselves, stand around wearing little but swimming trunks.

Whilst it would not be correct to call Frank Davison a 'loser' it is clear that many of his problems were self-generated and he too often let his enthusiasm get the better of him. With the *Reliance*, he got himself into the all-too-familiar trap of taking on something way beyond his means, aggravating the situation by refusing to acknowledge it and then allowing perfectionism to take over. Anybody who has known someone taking on the pleasure (and pain) of restoring or rejuvenating an old vessel will know of examples where the project, after a while, simply runs away from reality. Such people get too emotionally involved with the project, reason goes out of the window, costs mount up and the boat takes over. Once started, it is hard to leave a project half completed or, even harder, to know when to cut one's losses. This is what happened to Frank and Ann Davison.

But what could they have done? The bank which had a mortgage on the boat demanded its money back, then threatened to foreclose and sell it. Another creditor, to whom Frank owed only a small sum, took out a court summons which Frank could not honour. This would have led to a writ being nailed to the mast and the boat impounded. Whilst the bank dithered and took little action beyond threats, the other creditor got as far as obtaining a date for a court hearing. Ann and Frank knew that a forced sale would have raised barely enough to pay off the debts, leaving nothing for them.

No wonder then that they decided to clear out whilst they could. Before they left, Frank wrote a letter to his bank telling them they were leaving and heading for Cuba where they intended to sell *Reliance* to repay the loan. Frank believed this would maximise the amount they could realise. Nobody in England wanted a three quarter completed vessel. A successfully completed transatlantic voyage would surely have increased her value.

It was sheer bad luck that the Davison's ran into bad weather from day one and were unable to escape the English Channel. Had they met a fair wind, they surely would have made it into calmer and warmer waters and Frank was ingenious enough to have been able to complete the boat as they went along. Instead they met an inglorious end amid the rocky coves of the island of Portland, just underneath the lighthouse, swept there by the notorious tides of the Portland Race.

Enough has already been written about Donald Crowhurst's end. Hubris dragged him down and, once his courage failed him and he missed several opportunities to stop the whole charade, there was only one possible ending. Circumstances, not all of his making, certainly conspired against him. The withdrawal from the race of Bernard Moitessier and the sinking of Nigel Tetley's yacht *Victress* removed from Crowhurst any chance of his being able to slink home quietly, unnoticed and un-garlanded into some small Devon harbour in second or third position. This was irony of an exquisite degree. To have fraudulently set yourself up in a race which you then could not avoid winning would be too much for almost anyone, however strong, to face up to. Even a man as stable as Moitessier, who had nothing to answer for, could not face the thought of the adulation and exposure he knew would be awaiting him on his return to Europe and France. He turned his back on it all and disappeared into the islands of Polynesia 'to save my soul.'

Anyone who has seen the short video film made by the artist Tacita Dean of the wrecked and piteous *Teignmouth Electron* lying decaying on Cayman Brac with broken wings will appreciate the tragedy of the whole thing.

Angus Primrose's *Demon of Hamble* appears simply to have been overwhelmed by bad weather near the Bermuda triangle, during a period of equinoctial gales. There was little Primrose could have done to avoid his boat capsizing, taking on water and sinking. Such a possibility was inherent in the type of boat she was – a beamy, high freeboard, large volume hull with a big vulnerable centre cockpit.

What caused the loss of *Bucks Fizz* and her crew in the Fastnet race will never be known. Whilst multihulls have survived intact in weather worse than that experienced in the Irish Sea, the huge waves which built up so quickly were described by survivors as especially vicious. The fleet was in an area where the continental shelf shallows sharply and this ground effect is known to build up short steep seas not found in deeper waters. These seas, combined with a degree of inexperience on the part of Richard Pendred and his crew in leaving the centreboard lowered, may have contributed to the capsize. It will never be known whether all of the crew attempted to take to the life raft, but it was located nearby with only Richard Pendred inside. Many people have been lost (including Angus Primrose) in the very act of attempting to board a life raft and this may have been the reason for some or all of the crew's loss. Perhaps it would have been better had they stayed with the upturned vessel, as is generally considered best practice. *Bucks Fizz* would have floated high out of the water when inverted and I do know that the trimaran had an escape hatch in the underneath of the turtle deck wing. The crew would have been able to get in or out of the upturned hull and shelter inside waiting for rescue. This would have been uncomfortable, and wet, but probably safer than risking one's life in those seas in a small inflatable life raft. Many people all over the world have survived safely for long periods in upturned multihulls awaiting rescue. People have even survived in upturned monohulls for long periods. Most noticeably, Tony Bullimore survived in the Southern Ocean for five days trapped inside his upturned monohull, *Exide Challenger*, until rescued by the Australian Navy. He would never have survived in a life raft.

Manureva and Alain Colas were considered by many as an indestructible combination. They had circled the world twice, had crossed the Atlantic many times and had raced around the British Isles. What could go wrong on their last voyage together, a simple autumn sail from France to the Caribbean through mainly benign waters with a steady trade wind blowing from behind for much of the way? The weather in that year's Route de Rhum Race was generally favourable and *Manureva* disappeared south of the Azores where bad storms are rare. It is considered that the most likely reasons for the sudden disappearance of boat and skipper were either a collision with another ship or the trimaran breaking up and sinking from some inherent fault, possibly corrosion. Several people who saw the trimaran in St Malo before the start of the race commented that her aluminium structure was showing distinct signs of wear and corrosion. The three hulls were held together by four aluminium crossbeams each consisting of a number of tubes and struts. These were welded and bolted to each other and to the hulls. *Manureva* was 10 years old and had been built in a hurry in 1968, completed just in time for Tabarly to enter that year's OSTAR.

There are many problems in the welding and use of aluminium, including that of metal fatigue, not all visible to the naked eye. This would have been why Colas had the structure x-ray tested for corrosion before he left on his solo circumnavigation in 1973. Five years had elapsed since then and the boat had been sailed and pushed hard during that period for many thousands of miles. It is therefore quite likely that *Manureva* suffered a sudden and catastrophic failure which led to her breaking up and sinking before Colas could transmit a distress message.

Then there is the loss of *Three Cheers*. Was McMullen really in a fit state to undertake such a voyage only one day after he had buried his wife? Probably not, but I am sure nothing would have stopped him from going and the loss of Lizzie would have made him more determined than ever to win the race. He knew that he had a real chance of winning, knew his boat inside out, knew what she was capable of and he knew what he himself was capable of. He had been planning this race for four years and I do not believe that he would ever, for one moment, have considered pulling out. Those who knew Mike knew the determination he had when he had set his mind to do something.

The shortest route from Plymouth to Newport takes one right into the far North Atlantic where conditions are at their worst, with gales, icebergs and fog but where the distance to sail is the least. Most competitors make a compromise by taking a longer route further south in the hope of meeting better weather. In the first ever OSTAR Blondie Hasler (also an ex-marine) in his tiny junk rigged *Jester* sailed far to the north to Latitude 58° North and, if he had continued on a great circle route (i.e. the shortest route) from that position, he would have sailed right through the middle of Newfoundland. Hence Mike's assertion before the start that he might actually go so far north that he would sail behind the back of Newfoundland. This would have appealed to him in normal circumstances and after Lizzie's death he would have adopted an all-or-nothing approach to the race. I am sure he simply out sailed himself and his boat's capabilities and they either capsized or hit an iceberg or just broke up in big seas. Whatever happened, I like to believe that he was leading the fleet and enjoying every minute of it.

As for the others, well, a slip or a knock from a loose and swinging gaff can happen to anyone, even to the world's most experienced sailor. For that was what Tabarly was. He had spent virtually his whole life from 1964 to 1990, over 25 years, doing nothing but sail and race his boats over the oceans, often alone. Whilst he was ostensibly a French Naval Officer, the French Navy allowed him as much time off as he wanted and never engaged him in any real naval duties. But when it comes to it, even a man such as Tabarly can be taken off his guard and knocked overboard by an out of control spar, just like the most inexperienced of us.

Everybody inevitably relaxes when approaching harbour, when land is near and the wind and sea begin to calm down. This is when one is at ones most vulnerable. For the same reason, in the mountains more accidents have happened on descents after successful summit bids than during the ascents themselves. Both Rob James and Philip Walwyn were lost on the doorsteps of their destinations, James whilst entering Salcombe Harbour and Walwyn just 10 miles from Falmouth.

In James' case the cause of his loss was something as simple as a broken rope – the rope holding up the netting strung between the fore and aft crossbeams of his trimaran. Multihull sailors are used to jumping into and running over these nets without a thought.

Philip Walwyn, who was exhausted after a difficult voyage from the Azores, could simply have missed his footing (the boat did not have any guardrails or lifelines) but his family believe that he had a heart attack, collapsed and fell overboard and then had a further fatal attack as the rescue helicopter landed in Cornwall. That is the cause of death given on his death certificate. Philip had suffered from bad health for some years and hypothermia, caused from long immersion in the sea, is well known as being a trigger for a heart attack. But, as with Mike McMullen, Philip would have enjoyed himself to the last and had the satisfaction of all but completing one of the most amazing single-handed voyages of all. He was, I believe, the first man ever to sail an International 12 metre yacht, which normally has a crew of twelve or fourteen, solo across the Atlantic.

Finally, people have very strong opinions about Peter Tangvald. Many say he was totally irresponsible. He would set sail, often with only his young children on board, without regard to hurricanes, the season, pirates or other dangers. He ignored his own health problems and suffered the loss of two of his wives whilst at sea. His son, Thomas, recounts hearing his sister Carmen screaming from within *L'Artemis* as it broke up on the reef. This was probably the result of Peter's habit of locking his children into their cabins whilst at sea. If this was so, Carmen would have been unable to escape from the wreck before it was too late. Peter ignored pleas not to leave on his last voyage during the hurricane season or at the very least to take some crew with him.

Other people say he should be recognised as the superb seaman he was who sailed the seas for many years with simplicity, sincerity and skill and in an environmentally friendly way: something we should all admire. He was undoubtedly a fine seaman and navigator but he left a trail of loss and ruined lives behind him. People say a lot of what he wrote in his book, *At Any Cost*, is not true.

Here also was a man who suffered from ill health, experiencing heart problems all his life but he did not let this hinder him in his ambitions. He had a major heart attack a few years before his death when he was given merely a year to live. He suffered from angina and one must ask whether it was responsible for him to set off on his last voyage with only his young daughter on board and with his son being towed behind on his own boat. Thomas, who survived the accident, was never able to work out why his father ran onto the reef. Clare Allcard, who became Thomas's guardian, thinks it is likely that, during the voyage, Peter had another heart or angina attack (a used ampoule of nitro-glycerine was found amongst the wreckage) and in a befuddled state decided to keep well to windward of his destination so as not to miss the island entirely. He then misjudged his position and ran onto a reef which he thought he was well clear of. He had no one on board to help him apart from his young daughter.

As for Thomas Tangvald's disappearance in 2014, there can be no explanation. Here was a highly intelligent young man aged 37, at the height of his considerable powers, who left his wife and two young children ashore and embarked on what should have been an easy trip to look for a new home for them. Yet no sign of him or his boat has ever been found.

Thomas had a tragic life which is almost too unbearable to think about. He was born at sea, saw his mother shot by pirates, saw his step mother knocked overboard and drowned and who then saw his father and half-sister drown on a reef in the Caribbean. He then lost his own life at sea whilst on a simple single-handed passage.

All those who have been written about in this book were brave men and women doing what they loved most of all. We who knew them are poorer for their loss. Sailing is not a dangerous sport and, compared to mountaineering, losses are exceedingly rare. After all, to date over 200 people have died whilst trying to climb Mount Everest, of whom 18 died in 2015 alone and five have died so far in 2016. For every 100 climbers who have scaled K2, the world's second highest mountain, 29 have died – almost a one in three chance.

Nothing worth doing in this life is entirely free of risk and everyone who takes to the sea must be aware of this, however small the chance.

About the Author

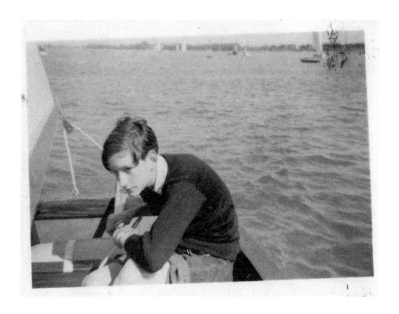

Nicholas Gray started sailing at the age of 6 on a small clinker-built scow in Chichester Harbour, progressing to sailing a Cadet, a Heron and a Firefly. During his school and university holidays he crewed on many yacht delivery trips crossing the Mediterranean and the Bay of Biscay several times.

He bought his first keelboat in 1967 – a small gaff cutter called

Roma, which was followed by two other wooden yachts.

In 1978 his sailing completely changed direction when he took part in the Two Handed Round Britain and Ireland Race in a friend's very fast but lightly built trimaran, sailing with Peter Phillips. They had to retire from that race, but he had caught the multihull bug and he bought a 35-foot bright yellow racing trimaran called *Whisky Jack* from Philip Walwyn, an old childhood friend, who features in this book.

In 1979 he took *Whisky Jack* into the 2,400 mile Azores and Back Race, putting up the fastest overall time and winning her class. In 1980, with Don Wood, he chartered the 56-foot trimaran *Great Britain IV*, which had won the 1978 Round Britain Race in the hands of Chay Blyth and Rob James. Nicholas and Don campaigned her for a year and intended to compete in the Two Handed Transatlantic Race the following year but decided she was not strong or seaworthy enough to survive a transatlantic race.

Next he bought a 30-foot trimaran, naming her *Applejack*, and she won her class in the 1982 Round Britain and Ireland Race.

More conventional yachts followed and he now owns a 42-foot classic wooden ketch which he keeps in Ramsgate and a 35-foot wooden motor yacht which he keeps on the Canal du Midi, in France.

Despite owning some 14 yachts and having raced against some of the top yachtsmen (many of whom feature in this book), Nicholas has never been a professional sailor. He has worked in Merchant Banking, as a solicitor and in the petroleum industry. He has also had an interest in a sailmaking company and owned a boatyard specialising in the restoration of classic wooden yachts.

Last Voyages is Nicholas' first book.

Acknowledgements

I would never have written this book, nor met many of the people featured, had my friend David Dillistone not introduced me to the somewhat dubious joys of racing his fragile and uncomfortable trimaran *Heretic* around the coasts of Britain and Ireland. This started my interest in the world of multihulls and in short-handed long-distance racing. Thank you, David.

Thanks must also go for the support I have had from all the people with whom I have sailed over the years, most importantly Peter Phillips, Julian Mustoe, Roger Hill and Don Wood.

I would also like to acknowledge the help and support I have had from Chris Waddington of Wicormarine, who kindly allowed me to clutter up his foreshore with a number of trimarans whilst they were in preparation for various voyages. Also many thanks for the invaluable advice I have received over the years from those knowledgeable gurus of all things 'maritime', Bob Brinton and Steve Parish.

I have had much assistance from author Clare Allcard (who gave me lots of encouragement and wise counsel in completing this my first book), from Edward Allcard, Denis Lochen of the Association Eric Tabarly, Jacqueline Tabarly, Susie Walwyn and her partner John Halsey, Kate Walwyn, Jill Blancaneaux,

Christina Pasquinucci, Guy Pendred, Colonel Tim Street (for information on 6 Metre yachts), Dan Primrose, Bob Comlay (for information on Bill Tilman and *En Avant*), John Lewis (Royal Western Yacht Club), Lester and Henrietta Barnes, Eve Lytton and Robert Bennett.

I would like to thank the publishers and authors of the books shown in bold in the bibliography which I have used as source material.

If any acknowledgements due to other authors and publishers have been inadvertently omitted I hope they will accept my apologies.

My thanks to everyone at Fernhurst Books and especially to Jeremy Atkins for being brave enough to take me on.

Finally, thank you to Josephine for everything (especially for putting up with my strange sailing exploits over the years).

Nicholas Gray
December 2016

Acknowledgements

Acknowledgement is gratefully made to the following publishers, authors, photographers and family members for permission to use material and photographs as follows:

Chapter 1: Frank & Ann Davison
Cover of *Last Voyage* by Ann Davison, published by William Heinemann.
Photo of *Reliance*: By kind permission of Weymouth Museum Trust.

Chapter 2: Donald Crowhurst
Photo of Donald Crowhurst: © Keystone Pictures USA / Alamy.
Photo of *Teignmouth Electron*: © geogphotos / Alamy

Chapter 3: Mike McMullen
Extracts from *Multihull Seamanship*: © Michael McMullen, 1976, *Multihull Seamanship*, Adlard Coles Nautical, an imprint of Bloomsbury Publishing Plc. By kind permission of Bloomsbury Publishing Plc.
Photos of Mike McMullen on board *Three Cheers*: © Ajax News & Feature Service / Alamy.

Chapter 4: Simon Richardson & Bill Tilman
Photos of *En Avant* & crew: taken by Sandy Lee, © the estate of W G Lee. By kind permission of Barbara Waite and Robert Lee.

Chapter 5: Alain Colas
Photo of Alain Colas: © Ajax News & Feature Service / Alamy.
Photo of *Manureva*: © Ajax News & Feature Service / Alamy.
Extracts from *The Atlantic Challenge*: © David Palmer, 1977, *The Atlantic Challenge*, Hollis & Carter. By kind permission of David Palmer.

Chapter 6: Richard Pendred
Photos of Richard Pendred and *Bucks Fizz*: By kind permission of Guy Pendred and the Pendred family archive.

Chapter 7: Angus Primrose
Photo of Angus Primrose and Blondie Hasler: © Ajax News & Feature Service / Alamy.
Photo of *Moody 33*: By kind permission of David Moody.

Last Voyages

Chapter 8: Rob James

Photos of Rob and Naomi James & *Colt Cars GB*: © Ajax News & Feature Service / Alamy.

Chapter 9: Peter & Thomas Tangvald

Extract and photos from *At Any Cost*: © Peter Tangvald, 1991, *At Any Cost*, Cruising Guide Publications. By kind permission of Christina Pasquinucci and Cruising Guide Publications.

Chapter 10: Eric Tabarly

Photo of Eric Tabarly: © Ajax News & Feature Service / Alamy.

Photos of *Pen Duick*: By kind permission of Denis Lochen of the Association of Eric Tabarly.

Chapter 11: Philip Walwyn

Photos of Philip and *Kate*: From the Walwyn family archive. By kind permission of Kate Walwyn, Susie Walwyn and John Halsey.

About the Author

Photo of Nicholas Gray as a boy: From the author's family archive.

Every effort has been made to contact the copyright holders of the extracts and photographs used in this book. If any errors or omissions have inadvertently been made, they will be rectified in future editions provided that written notification is made to the publishers.

Bibliography

Allcard, Clare, 1994, *A Gypsy Life*. Ashford, Buchan & Enright.

Allcard, Clare, 1990, *The Intricate Art of Living Afloat*. W W Norton & Co.

Allcard, Edward, 1967, *Voyage Alone*. Robert Hale.

Allcard, Edward, 1950, *Single Handed Passage*. Putnam & Co Ltd.

Allcard, Edward, 1952, *Temptress Returns*. Putnam & Co Ltd.

Anderson, J R L, 1980, ***High Mountains & Cold Seas***. Victor Gollanz Ltd.

Boehmer, Richard, 1977, *Multihull Ocean Racing*. Boehmer Publishing.

Borden, C A, 1968, ***Sea Quest***. Robert Hale Ltd.

Chichester, Francis, 1967, *Gipsy Moth Circles the World*. Hodder & Stoughton.

Colas, Alain, 1978, ***Around the World Alone***. Barron's Educational Series Inc.

Davison, Ann, 1953, ***Last Voyage***. William Heinemann.

Davison, Ann, 1956, *My Ship Is So Small*. Peter Davies Ltd.

Eakin, Chris, 2009, ***A Race Too Far***. Ebury Press

Foster, Lloyd, 1989, ***OSTAR***. Haynes Publishing Group.

Holm, Donald, 1975, ***The Circumnavigators***. Angus & Robertson.

Gardner, L T, 1979, ***Fastnet '79***. George Godwin Ltd.

Illingworth, John, 1949, *Offshore*. Robert Ross & Co Ltd.

Illingworth, John, 1972, ***The Malham Story***. Nautical Publishing Company

James, Naomi, 1979, *At One with the Sea*. Stanley Paul.

James, Naomi, 1987, ***Courage at Sea***. Stanley Paul.

James, Rob, 1983, ***Multihulls Offshore***. Macmillan London Ltd.

Knox-Johnston, Robin, 1969, *A World of My Own*. Cassel & Co Ltd.

Lockley, R M, 1930, *Dream Island*. H F & G Witherby.

Lockley, R M, 1934, *Island Days*. H F & G Witherby

Last Voyages

Lockley, R M, 1947, *Letters from Skokholm*. J M Dent & Sons Ltd.

Madge, Tim, 1995, **The Last Hero**. Hodder & Stoughton.

McMullen, Michael, 1971, *A Cruise in Company Binkie in the Round Britain Race*. Roving Commisisons No. 11 RCC Press Ltd

McMullen Michael, 1975, *Three Cheers for the Hebrides*. RCC Journal 1975 RCC Press Ltd.

McMullen, Michael, 1976, **Multihull Seamanship**. Nautical Publishing Co Ltd.

Nicholls, Peter, 2001, **A Voyage for Madmen**. Profile Books Ltd.

Page, Frank, 1972 **Solo to America**. Adlard Coles Ltd

Page, Frank, 1980, **Alone Against the Atlantic**. The Observer Ltd.

Palmer, David, 1977, *The Atlantic Challenge - The Story of the Trimaran FT*. Hollis & Carter.

Reneham, Edward, 2016, *Desperate Voyage*. New Street Communications LLC.

Richardson, Dorothy, 1986, **The Quest of Simon Richardson**. Victor Gollancz.

Southby-Tailyour, E, 1998, *Blondie*. Perr & Sword Books Ltd.

Tabarly, Eric, 1971, **Pen Duick**. Adlard Coles Ltd.

Tabarly, Eric, 2010, **Memories of the Open Sea**. Sports Books Ltd.

Tangvald, Peter, 1996, **Sea Gypsy**. William Kimber & Co Ltd.

Tangvald, Peter, 1991, **At Any Cost, Love, Life and Death at Sea**. Cruising Guide Publications.

Tetley, Nigel, 1970, **Trimaran Solo**. Nautical Publishing Company.

Tilman, H W, 1987, *The Eight Sailing/Mountain-Exploration Books*. Diadem Books Ltd.

Tilman, H W, 1974, **Ice With Everything**. Nautical Publishing Co Ltd.

Tomalin, Nicholas and Hall, Ron, 1970, **The Strange Voyage of Donald Crowhurst**. Hodder and Stoughton.

Weld, Philip, 1982, *Moxie, The American Challenge*. The Bodley Head.

Other titles you might be interested in...

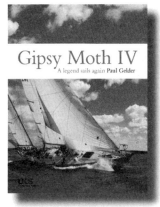

Gipsy Moth IV
Paul Gelder
The definitive history of a sailing icon.
A beautifully illustrated book telling the
remarkable story of Gipsy Moth's rise, fall
and triumphant rise again. With exclusive
photographs of the boat, the restoration
project and dramatic images from both of
her epic voyages.

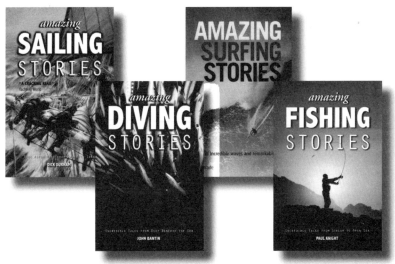

The Amazing Stories series
Treasure troves of tales of adventure from the worlds of sailing, surfing,
diving and fishing. Each is packed with accounts of exploits, triumphs
and disasters from across centuries and around the globe.

🐟 FERNHURST BOOKS

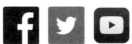
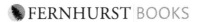